SUPPLEMENTAL HEALTH INSURANCE

The Health Insurance Association of America
Washington, DC 20004-1109

© 1998 by the Health Insurance Association of America
All rights reserved. Published 1998
Printed in the United States of America

ISBN 1-879143-42-9

TABLE OF CONTENTS

FIGURES AND TABLES... v

FOREWORD... vii

PREFACE ix

ACKNOWLEDGMENTS xi

ABOUT THE AUTHORS.. xiii

Chapter 1
INTRODUCTION TO SUPPLEMENTAL HEALTH
INSURANCE PRODUCTS.. 1

Chapter 2
MEDICARE SUPPLEMENTS 29

Chapter 3
HOSPITAL INDEMNITY COVERAGE 63

Chapter 4
SPECIFIED DISEASE INSURANCE.. 83

Chapter 5
ACCIDENT COVERAGE... 101

Chapter 6
DENTAL PLANS 123

Chapter 7
SPECIALTY PLANS 145

Chapter 8
THE SUPPLEMENTAL HEALTH INSURANCE MARKET.................. 165

Appendix A
INDIVIDUAL ACCIDENT AND SICKNESS INSURANCE
MINIMUM STANDARDS ACT... 171

Appendix B
MODEL REGULATION TO IMPLEMENT THE INDIVIDUAL
ACCIDENT AND SICKNESS INSURANCE MINIMUM
STANDARDS ACT 177

Appendix C
MEDICARE SUPPLEMENT INSURANCE MINIMUM STANDARDS
MODEL ACT 213

Appendix D
RULES GOVERNING ADVERTISEMENTS OF ACCIDENT AND
SICKNESS INSURANCE WITH INTERPRETIVE GUIDELINES 219

Appendix E
DISCLOSURE STATEMENT FOR MEDICARE BENEFICIARIES 245

NOTES 247

SUGGESTED READINGS 251

GLOSSARY 253

INDEX 273

FIGURES AND TABLES

CHAPTER 2

Figure
Figure 2.1 . . . . Rating by Medicare Beneficiaries of Health Care Quality, Health, and Health Care Costs

Tables
Table 2.1 . . . . History of Medicare Components
Table 2.2 . . . . Medicare (Part A) Hospital Services—Per Benefit Period
Table 2.3 . . . . Medicare (Part B) Medical Services—Per Calendar Year
Table 2.4 . . . . Ten Standard Medicare Supplement Plans and Sales Distribution

CHAPTER 5

Table
Table 5.1 . . . . Costs of Unintentional Injuries in the United States, 1995

CHAPTER 6

Figures
Figure 6.1 . . . . Dental Care Costs: Source of Payment, 1994
Figure 6.2 . . . . Dental Plans by Employer Size

Tables
Table 6.1 . . . . Sample Dental Benefits
Table 6.2 . . . . Sample Frequency of Dental Services

FOREWORD

The HIAA Insurance Education Program aims to be the leader in providing the highest quality educational material and service to the health insurance industry and other related health care fields.

To accomplish this mission, the Program seeks to fulfill the following goals:

1. Provide a tool for use by member company personnel to enhance quality and efficiency of services to the public;
2. Provide a career development vehicle for employees and other health care industry personnel; and
3. Further general understanding of the role and contribution of the health insurance industry to the financing, administration, and delivery of health care services.

The Insurance Education Program provides the following services:

1. A comprehensive course of study in the fundamentals of health insurance, long-term care insurance, disability income insurance, managed care, medical expense insurance, health care fraud, and supplemental health insurance;
2. Certificate by examination of educational achievement for all courses;
3. Programs to recognize accomplishment in the industry and academic communities through course evaluation and certification, which enables participants to obtain academic or continuing education credits; and
4. Development of educational, instructional, training, and informational materials related to the health insurance and health care industries.

PREFACE

Even though most people are covered by traditional private or public medical insurance in the United States, the need for supplemental health insurance is great. More than an estimated 85 million people carry at least one type of supplemental product. Supplemental health insurance is offered by health insurance companies to give insureds protection against risk in addition—or as a supplement—to what their medical insurance provides.

Students of Health Insurance Association of America (HIAA) courses were introduced to the concepts underlying supplemental health insurance in *Fundamentals of Health Insurance: Part A* and *Fundamentals of Health Insurance: Part B*. The purpose of this new textbook, *Supplemental Health Insurance*, is to provide more specific information on the major supplemental products in the marketplace: Medicare supplement; hospital indemnity policies; specified disease insurance; accident coverage; dental coverage; and specialty plans, including prescription drug insurance, vision insurance, and TRICARE supplement. The gaps in health coverage that lead to the need for additional insurance are discussed for each insurance product.

The book opens with an introductory chapter describing supplemental insurance products, and concludes with a look at the supplemental market.

The contents of this book are educational, not a statement of policy. The views expressed or suggested in this and all other HIAA textbooks are those of the contributing authors or editors. They are not necessarily the opinions of the HIAA or of its member companies.

ACKNOWLEDGMENTS

Chapter 1: Introduction to Supplemental Health Insurance Products
Steven E. Lippai
Combined Insurance Company of America

Chapter 2: Medicare Supplements
John A. Boni
Physicians Mutual Insurance Company

Chapter 3: Hospital Indemnity Coverage
Ken Smith
Mutual of Omaha Insurance Company

Carol Ashton-Hergenhan
Karen L. Fleming
Union Fidelity Life Insurance Company

Chapter 4: Specified Disease Insurance
Claire W. Yarborough
John Garrison
Colonial Life & Accident Insurance Company

Chapter 5: Accident Coverage
Milton Gary Hickman
J.C. Penney Life Insurance Company

Chapter 6: Dental Plans
Eric S. Waters
Principal Financial Group

Chapter 7: Specialty Plans
Darcy Duesenberg
Amy Friedman
Michelle Lebens
Mutual of Omaha Insurance Company

James R. Latham
USAA Life Insurance Company

Chapter 8: The Supplemental Health Insurance Market
John A. Boni
Physicians Mutual Insurance Company

Reviewers
Shannon M. Anderson
Health Insurance Association of America

Bruce Boyd
Bruce Boyd Associates

Marianne Miller
Health Insurance Association of America

Editor
Jane J. Stein
The Stein Group

ACKNOWLEDGMENTS

Chapter 1: Introduction to Supplemental Health Insurance Products
Steven E. Lippai
Combined Insurance Company of America

Chapter 2: Medicare Supplements
John A. Boni
Physicians Mutual Insurance Company

Chapter 3: Hospital Indemnity Coverage
Ken Smith
Mutual of Omaha Insurance Company

Carol Ashton-Hergenhan
Karen L. Fleming
Union Fidelity Life Insurance Company

Chapter 4: Specified Disease Insurance
Claire W. Yarborough
John Garrison
Colonial Life & Accident Insurance Company

Chapter 5: Accident Coverage
Milton Gary Hickman
J.C. Penney Life Insurance Company

Chapter 6: Dental Plans
Eric S. Waters
Principal Financial Group

Chapter 7: Specialty Plans
Darcy Duesenberg
Amy Friedman
Michelle Lebens
Mutual of Omaha Insurance Company

James R. Latham
USAA Life Insurance Company

Chapter 8: The Supplemental Health Insurance Market
John A. Boni
Physicians Mutual Insurance Company

Reviewers
Shannon M. Anderson
Health Insurance Association of America

Bruce Boyd
Bruce Boyd Associates

Marianne Miller
Health Insurance Association of America

Editor
Jane J. Stein
The Stein Group

ABOUT THE AUTHORS

Carol Ashton-Hergenhan has held several management positions at Union Fidelity Life Insurance Company and currently is responsible for corporate communications. For more than 15 years, Ashton-Hergenhan has served as a member of the board of a private psychiatric hospital, an acute medical/surgical hospital, and a regional health system.

John A. Boni has enjoyed a 21-year career in insurance sales and marketing—beginning as an agent and advancing to product management. Currently, Boni is a design analyst at Physicians Mutual Insurance Company where his responsibilities include the development of individual and group life and health insurance products.

Darcy Duesenberg is a customer relations consultant at Mutual of Omaha. She has over eight years of experience at Mutual with customer service in support of managed care and prescription drug programs. She is currently responsible for supporting 19 HMO, preferred provider, and indemnity prescription drug programs. Duesenberg has been instrumental in the expansion of prescription drug services, the implementation of point-of-service products, and HMO site development.

Karen L. Fleming currently serves as associate counsel and assistant secretary at Union Fidelity Life Insurance Company where she is responsible for legal matters related to the company's product development and marketing. Her responsibilities include overseeing regulatory actions and compliance issues for products marketed through direct response sales techniques.

Amy Friedman is a clinical pharmacist at Mutual of Omaha where she is involved with formulary management, drug information, disease state management, and pharmacotherapy consultation services. Friedman has clinical experience in hospital pharmacy practice, teaching, and collaboration with physicians and other health care professionals to optimize patient drug therapy.

John Garrison is assistant vice president and counsel of government relations at Colonial Life & Accident Insurance Company, where his responsibilities include development and advocacy in legislative matters at the state and federal levels. Previously, Garrison held positions in the legislative and judicial branches of the government.

Milton Gary Hickman is associate actuary for the J.C. Penney Insurance Group. For 14 years, he specialized in financial analysis of direct response techniques and studied marketing segmentation, modeling, appraisal, and capital management. He is a fellow of the Society of Actuaries and a member of the American Academy of Actuaries.

James R. Latham is currently assistant vice president for health insurance services at USAA Life Insurance Company and has been associated with the health insurance industry for 25 years. While with Blue Cross and Blue Shield of Massachusetts, Latham was responsible for overseeing CHAMPUS and Medicare Part B programs.

Michelle Lebens is a regional contracting specialist at Mutual of Omaha where she is developing and expanding preferred provider, point-of-service, and HMO provider networks in the midwest. A marketing professional with 15 years of experience, Lebens has also worked in product development and sales administration.

Steven E. Lippai specializes in supplemental accident and health insurance in the United States, Canada, and the United Kingdom. He has served on several committees of the Health Insurance Association of America and the American Academy of Actuaries and is senior vice president and actuary for Combined Insurance Company of America.

Ken Smith is product manager of supplemental health products at Mutual of Omaha. In his 20-year career in the industry, Smith has held a variety of sales and marketing positions and specifically directed his attention to product management and development. He is currently a member of HIAA's Supplemental Insurance Committee.

Eric S. Waters is currently a market director for the Principal Financial Group. He oversees claims, contracts, and underwriting for dental, disability, life, and vision products and is accountable for growth and profitability of group nonmedical products in the state of Florida. Waters has completed several HIAA education courses.

Claire W. Yarborough is vice president for compliance and government relations for Colonial Life & Accident Insurance Company. She oversees regulatory matters including compliance and market conduct and acts as liaison with state and federal officials. She is a current member and former chair of the HIAA's Supplemental Insurance Committee.

Chapter 1

INTRODUCTION TO SUPPLEMENTAL HEALTH INSURANCE PRODUCTS

1 *Introduction*
2 *Supplemental Health Insurance Market*
5 *Classifying Supplemental Products*
14 *Market Characteristics of the Purchaser*
15 *General Product Characteristics*
19 *Overview of Supplemental Products*
27 *Summary*
27 *Key Terms*

■ Introduction

supplement—Something added to complete a thing, make up for a deficiency, or extend or strengthen the whole.

This definition from *The American Heritage Dictionary of the English Language, Third Edition,* provides great insight into the reason for the existence and popularity of the many forms of supplemental health insurance. Simply stated, many consumers feel a strong need to buy supplemental insurance since it makes their health insurance more complete. It extends their existing health insurance or employee benefit program by providing additional protection at an affordable cost against the risks that concern them the most. Moreover, the products that fall within this classification are readily available and easily purchased.

The supplemental insurance marketplace plays a role that goes beyond just filling the needs of today's consumers. It provides insurance carriers with a vehicle for developing new health insurance markets. For example, the nursing home insurance products of the 1970s were considered supplemental health insurance. These products only provided coverage for skilled nursing care following a hospitalization. As insurance companies became more comfortable with this risk, the coverage was gradually expanded. Today, nursing home insurance products have evolved into long-term care insurance—a product that stands on its own. (It has its own HIAA textbook—*Long-Term Care: Knowing the Risk, Paying the Price*—and so is not covered by this book.) Dental and vision insurance currently are considered part of the supplemental insurance marketplace, although increasingly they are incorporated within basic group health plans.

This book covers the supplemental health insurance products that exist today. It begins with this introductory chapter, which describes the many different products that are available today to consumers and explores the consumer needs that are satisfied by each type of product. A brief description of the main types of supplemental products and the size of the market served also is included.

The remaining chapters of this book provide detailed information about each of the six main product types that are generally considered as supplemental health insurance. These are Medicare supplements, hospital indemnity coverage, specified disease products, accident coverage, dental plans, and specialty plans (including prescription drugs, vision, and TRICARE [formerly the Civilian Health and Medical Program of the Uniformed Services, or CHAMPUS] supplements). The specific consumer needs that are met by each type as well as information concerning the methods for both distributing and administering the product are discussed. The typical benefit structures, characteristics of the premium rating structures, and regulatory considerations also are reviewed for each product. The final chapter considers the future of the supplemental insurance market.

■ Supplemental Health Insurance Market

The supplemental health insurance market contains an array of products that are distributed to customers in a variety of ways in a competitive market. Insurance agents and brokers often sell individual products directly to the consumer. The agency distribution system is comprised of sales people who are under contract to an insurance company through a management arrangement. These sales people may be either agents or brokers. Agents may be employees of either the insurer or the agency for which they work, although most agents are independent contractors. The agent does the actual selling and also is critical in field underwriting, policyholder service, and public relations.

A company may, in addition to or instead of agents and brokers, sell supplemental health insurance through mass marketing as a way to reach a large number of prospects simultaneously. Some mass marketing techniques include direct mail, association third-party sponsorship, vending machines, and over-the-counter sales.

The fastest growing distribution site is the customer's place of employment. Work site efforts are offered through the employer and are designed to augment the employer's benefit package. They may consist of group voluntary products for which employees complete an enrollment form after reviewing descriptive brochures. Alternatively, this distribution approach may use individual products for which employees complete the application with the help of an enroller who personally describes the available insurance options during business hours.

Supplemental products also are offered through the Internet. Several insurance companies and insurance agents have Web sites that supply potential customers with information about insurance needs, supplemental products, and rates.

It is difficult to determine the total size of the supplemental health insurance market. Often these coverages are added to basic products as riders. For example, it is possible to add accidental death riders or critical illness riders for specified diseases to life insurance policies. These riders usually are not counted in any product survey. In addition, employer group policies may be self-administered and report only premiums and not a tabulation of covered lives. Even when the number of lives is reported, that number usually represents only insured employees and not insured family members.

Another problem in determining the size of the market is that there is a variety of sources for this information, and each source may compile the data differently.

SUPPLEMENTAL HEALTH INSURANCE

Given these caveats, however, it is safe to say that over $20 billion of annual premium is written each year, providing coverage for more than 85 million people. It is important to realize that individuals having more than one supplemental coverage may be counted more than once.

Medicare supplement products are the most popular of all the supplemental coverages. Nearly 85 percent of all people aged 65 and older have Medicare supplement products to provide coverage over and above what Medicare provides and/or pays for.[1] About 80 percent of the market is supplied by 25 insurance carriers. The market is relatively evenly split among products supplied by Blue Cross organizations, products marketed to associations and other affinity groups, and individual policies sold directly to consumers. The total premium volume of Medicare supplement insurance in 1995 was $12.5 billion. Approximately $8.6 billion of premium was on individual policies, with the remaining $3.9 billion on group policy forms.

The second most popular supplement in terms of premium sales is accident-only coverages with more than $2.2 billion of premium, according to a survey of supplemental insurance conducted by the HIAA of 95 member companies.[2] Accident-only policies usually cover expenses only related to a specific accident. Since the average premium for an accident-only policy is about one-tenth the premium of a Medicare supplement policy, the popularity of these coverages in terms of the number of people insured is quite significant. It has been estimated that more than 30 million people have accident-only supplemental insurance, which ranges from on-the-job accident policies purchased by employers for their employees to single flight insurance sold at airports. At least 35 insurance companies actively offer it on a group basis, and more than 80 companies offer it using individual products.

Dental insurance, which provides coverage of preventive as well as corrective procedures, is the next most popular supplemental product, producing approximately $1.7 billion of annual premium. Approximately 40 companies offer this product, mostly on a group basis. That does not include the supplemental dental programs that are part of managed care plans such as health maintenance organizations (HMOs) or self-insured group medical trusts. Including this broader universe, dental coverage could rank as the second-largest supplemental product line.

4

Following these three products, the next most popular supplemental plans are specified disease coverages such as cancer insurance, which provides benefits only for expenses associated with cancer, and hospital indemnity plans, which provide daily benefits for hospitalization. According to the HIAA Supplemental survey, these policies generated $1.1 billion and $0.8 billion of annual premium, respectively. Approximately 65 companies offer specified disease policies, and more than 100 companies market hospital indemnity programs. Most of this coverage is written on individual policies.

Classifying Supplemental Products

Health insurance is a broad array of coverages providing for the payment of benefits for losses from medical expense, accident, disability, and accidental death and dismemberment. Consumers purchase health insurance, both basic and supplemental, for a wide variety of reasons. Some products provide protection for the cost of health care. This protection is often considered a necessity. The universal need for this protection is one of the forces that periodically drives the call for health care reform. Other health insurance is purchased to provide protection for the risks of reduced earnings or diminished financial resources in case of illness or injury.

The basic (nonsupplemental) coverage purchased either as part of an employee group or by an individual rarely provides total coverage. There are almost always significant gaps. For example, medical products for both groups and individuals have deductibles, coinsurance, and benefit maximums. Even managed care plans have copayments and limitations on the health care providers that can be used. In addition, sick leave programs may only be available to certain classes of employees, and disability programs have benefit elimination periods and eligibility waiting periods.

Few employers can afford to make their group programs so comprehensive that they cover all possible insurance needs for all of their employees. As the cost of benefit programs continues to rise, employers increasingly are requiring their employees to assume more of the risk. While the vast majority of the common risks are protected through a

SUPPLEMENTAL HEALTH INSURANCE

group's benefit package, each employee has unique individual or family situations.

For people purchasing individual insurance, some types of basic individual products may be unavailable due to a person's age, occupation, or risk profile. Basic disability income protection may not be affordable for many consumers.

There are other situations in which people with group or individual health insurance may find themselves exposed to risks not covered by the basic insurance package. There could be special health-related needs for one or more family members. Also, risk-averse individuals may never feel that all their insurance needs are adequately covered by their basic insurance. Supplemental insurance can fill all these gaps.

It is important to realize that each individual has a different perception of risk and may be more or less risk averse than another person. The perception of risk often comes from a personal experience that occurred to the individual, a family member, or a close friend. Risk also may be related to the ability of the individual to absorb the financial impact of an accident or illness by using existing savings and available basic insurance protection.

Supplemental insurance policies are designed, priced, and sold to serve as a supplement to individual or family basic health needs. Supplemental insurance benefits are paid generally to the insured, who has the discretion to determine how they will be used. Typically, benefits are used for three purposes:

- to cover medical costs (doctor, hospital, clinics, drugs, tests, etc.) not covered by primary coverage; and
- to cover related costs (travel, lodging, counseling, etc.) that would not have been incurred but for the illness or injury; and
- to cover lost income that would not have been missing but for the illness or injury.

Supplemental Coverage of Medical Expenses

Basic health care coverages are intended to directly reimburse the insured or the provider for the actual expenses incurred for health care necessary to restore or maintain a person's health to a level that is generally accepted by the medical community as appropriate for the individual's age and health history. Supplemental products in this category expand coverages, fill gaps in benefits, or fill specific short-term needs.

Types of Supplemental Medical Expense Products

Expanding the types of conditions insured. Dental and vision insurance are two examples of this type of supplemental product. Most basic medical plans only provide dental coverage due to injury. Vision coverage is provided either for injury or when a specific medical condition such as glaucoma or a cataract is present. Supplemental dental insurance extends coverage by providing for the cost of routine dental exams, common dental treatments, and oral appliances. Supplemental vision insurance extends coverage by providing for the cost of routine eye exams and corrective lenses.

Filling the gaps. Medicare supplement insurance is designed to fill the gaps of government-provided health care insurance for seniors by increasing the number of days of in-hospital coverage and by covering deductibles, coinsurance, and any excess charges. It also can expand managed care coverage by providing for the cost of treatment during foreign travel, at-home recovery, preventive medical care, and prescription drugs. Some of these benefits are contained within all of the standardized Medicare supplement policies while other benefits are optional.

A variation of Medicare supplement insurance is provided by Medicare SELECT contracts. These policies cover expenses incurred for medical services provided by a specific network of health care providers. Premiums for these policies tend to be lower than for the standardized plans. However, the only coverage for out-of-network care is generally for emergency treatment.

Covering specific short-term needs. Some products provide for the cost of medical care for short-term needs, such as for participation in athletic events or for the rescue, evacuation, and medical treatment of hikers, mountain climbers, or skiers. Another short-term product provides for health care coverages for Americans traveling abroad or foreign visitors in the United States. Generally the term of the insurance for this type of supplemental coverage extends only as long as the event being covered.

The Need for Supplemental Coverage of Medical Expenses

The value in supplemental health insurance comes from the consumer's perception of the risk involved. Caring for an unwell individual—a parent, for example, or child—is universally accepted as the proper, morally correct thing to do. In the United States, the extension of life for a family member, even for a few weeks or months, is often done at any cost, even if it means spending much of a family's financial resources.

Supplemental health insurance, such as Medicare supplement policies, are seen as a way to absorb the potentially high costs of treatment of the often life-threatening illnesses that can accompany old age. Among that population, there are just too many possible medical catastrophes with large financial impacts to be ignored.

It is worth noting that the American approach to using high-cost treatments is unique. Perhaps this cultural situation is the result of having access to the most up-to-date medical technology in the world. Or perhaps it is the belief that everyone should have the very best opportunity for good health and long life. In many other countries, the rationing of health care resources is a function of the national health programs.

For example, kidney failure is one of the most common physical occurrences prior to the death of an elderly person. In many ways, it is just part of the natural process of dying. However, it is possible to treat kidney failure by dialysis. In Germany, kidney dialysis is rare for anyone over the age of 70. In the United States, it is the commonly accepted treatment for everyone at any age.

There are numerous examples of medical treatments that have an impact on people of all ages. Heart surgery is much more common today than even five years ago. Gene therapy may offer medical possibilities not thought of until recently. Because so many Americans believe they have the right to even the most expensive forms of medical care, they are willing to prepare for the need for such care by purchasing supplemental insurance.

While some types of supplemental health care coverages are designed to provide for catastrophic medical situations such as the ones described above, other types are constructed to assist families with the more routine types of care needed to maintain health. Dental and vision insurance fall into this category. Here the maximum benefits are relatively low. However, by having this type of insurance the consumer is encouraged to seek the frequent, routine care that minimizes the need for more extensive and more expensive work. These coverages provide an easy way for budgeting payments for appropriate care. More importantly, the coverage often includes access to a network of qualified dental or vision care providers who offer their services at a discount over the standard retail price structure, thereby offering the insured more services at lower cost than he/she might otherwise be able to obtain.

Prescription drug insurance also gives the insured access to lower cost services through discounts that are available for generic drugs or for drugs purchased in large quantities by mail.

Supplemental Coverage of Related Expenses

Many accidents and illnesses create significant financial burdens that can greatly affect the life-style of the person or family involved. Many supplemental policies provide cash benefits for people who have experienced an accident or a long-term or costly illness. These benefits cover related expenses and lost income while a person is disabled or hospitalized. There is no direct tie to the medical expenses incurred except that the cash benefit is paid when a specific medical event occurs. It is then up to the discretion of the insured to apply these benefits toward the payment of related expenses (those costs, both medical and nonmedical in nature, that would not have been incurred but for the accident or sickness) and to replace lost income.

The level of cash benefit the insured selects depends upon the extent to which the insured is willing to either accept a lower standard of living or self-insure the contingency. Self-insurance usually means relying on savings, family, or friends to supply the necessary financial help.

Types of Supplemental Coverage for Related Expenses

One of the most common uses of supplemental health insurance is to provide an income in case the insured is sick or disabled and unable to work. Many people work for companies that do not have short-term sick leave or disability programs, and they get paid only when they work. There are, however, numerous situations that could create an inability to work. Hospital indemnity insurance and accident-only disability insurance are two types of supplemental insurance products that can be used to meet this need.

Other supplemental products cover nonmedical expenses related to an accident or sickness. For example, if an insured needs specialized treatment at a medical facility that is a long distance from home, travel expenses for the insured and family members may be incurred. Or family members may need to reduce the amount of time they can spend working to care for the insured while he/she is recovering at home. Other expenses may be incurred for structural modifications at home after a crippling stroke or paralysis due to an accident. The cost of installing ramps or wheelchair lifts and making bathrooms, kitchens, or automobiles accessible is not reimbursable through any basic medical insurance program. Supplemental health insurance products that may provide these types of benefits include specified disease coverages, such as cancer or critical illness insurance, and personal accident insurance plans.

The Need for Coverage of Related Expenses

Supplemental protection is needed to help individuals and families recover from (a) the loss of income due to an accident or sickness beyond that provided by a basic disability policy or (b) the additional nonmedical expenses that accompany a serious injury or illness. In most cases it extends an individual's coverage to areas not included in the basic insurance or employee benefit package.

Income replacement supplements. The need to use supplemental accident and health products for basic income replacement probably is much greater than most insurance professionals realize. According to the Employee Benefits Research Institute, 48 percent of all nonfarm workers who are employed by private employers do not have short-term sick leave programs.[3] This surprisingly large number was confirmed by another recent study that indicated that 50 percent of all workers in the private sector do not have sick leave coverage.[4]

This information indicates that many people only get paid when they work, and they either work when they have a minor injury or illness, or they stay at home for the shortest period of time possible. Obviously, they cannot work while they are confined in the hospital. And a condition that requires a hospital stay may also be serious enough to involve a lengthy convalescence period at home while they recover.

Hospital indemnity coverage has a significant appeal to people concerned about the risk of losing their income after becoming hospitalized. The daily benefits can be at a level roughly equivalent to the income lost by the insured. Even benefits for family members can be viewed as replacing lost income since a spouse or parent may not go to work full time so that he/she can be with the sick family member. For the 50 percent of the private sector employees who do not have sick leave, it would be desirable to have hospital indemnity coverage, low-cost supplemental insurance that provides protection against the loss of income in specific situations involving certain serious injuries or illnesses.

Traditional disability income products may fulfill the income replacement need in a more complete way. However, these products often are not available or not affordable for many workers. Traditional income replacement products generally are sold using extensive financial and physical underwriting, which can be costly and also exclude certain high-risk populations. Supplemental disability plans generally have less restricted underwriting.

Regardless of the effects of underwriting, income replacement plans may still not be available to all persons seeking disability protection. They generally are not available to part-time workers or employees in certain occupations.

SUPPLEMENTAL HEALTH INSURANCE

Even if the coverage is available, traditional disability income protection may not be affordable for those with moderate incomes. For example, the medium income for a family of four in the United States is approximately $40,000. To insure the net, after-tax income, a skilled blue-collar tradesperson such as a plumber or carpenter may have to spend $1,500, or almost 4 percent of his/her annual salary, to obtain coverage that would begin after a 30-day elimination period and have a maximum benefit period of only five years. The costs would be higher for people in riskier occupations and lower for supervisors and office workers. Most families with a $40,000 income would find it difficult to spend $1,500 insuring their income because it would consume too great a portion of their limited financial resources. As a result, such coverage often is not purchased.

Besides hospital indemnity insurance, accident-only disability insurance is a supplemental product that can provide short-term loss-of-income protection. The comparatively low cost of the accident-only product is attractive to many individuals. Also, coverage often is provided from the first day of disability, a factor that naturally has appeal to the large portion of workers without sick leave.

For young employees who are rarely sick or for healthy older workers, the appeal of accident-only disability insurance is quite great. It provides coverage for the unexpected accident while keeping overall cost at an affordable level. Many people who keep themselves in good health do not see a need to spend the extra dollars necessary for sickness coverage. Although it may seem like a waste of money to buy something that will go unused, nevertheless, each year, according to the National Safety Council, 19.3 million people are disabled for more than one day from an injury.[5]

Supplemental coverage for related expenses. The financial consequences of an accident or illness often extend beyond the loss of income and beyond the medical costs of the hospitals, physicians, and treatments. When one family member receives medical treatment, additional expenses may be incurred, such as living expenses while away from home, child care, transportation, and household help. In addition, it is often important for a family member to take time off from work to act as a caregiver during the recovery period.

INTRODUCTION TO SUPPLEMENTAL HEALTH INSURANCE PRODUCTS

When hospitalization is involved, family members want to be nearby. They often spend extensive periods at the hospital. They travel to the hospital every day. They incur expenses related to travel, eating their meals away from home, and, if they have children, child care costs. Sometimes, additional living expenses are incurred because a family member wants to be very close to the hospital at all times. In this situation, he/she may take up temporary residence in a motel nearby the medical facility. This can happen if the patient requires specialized care that is best received at a regional hospital or even if the household is located more than one or two hours away from the local hospital.

The impact on a family of a serious illness or injury can be tremendous, and a study of more than 2,100 families of patients who had been treated for one of nine serious illnesses, such as acute respiratory failure, severe congestive heart failure, and metastatic lung or colon cancer, clearly illustrates this impact.[6] Each of the nine conditions was associated with an expected six-month mortality rate between 30 and 70 percent. In other words, the conditions were quite serious. Results of this study indicated that one-third of the patients required considerable care giving from a family member. The severe caregiver burdens reported by families included the need to make major life changes to care for the patient and the inability to function normally because of the stress of the illness. Slightly less than a third (31 percent) of the families reported losing most of their savings. A smaller portion (29 percent) reported losing their major source of household income. At least one major adverse impact requiring something other than caregiver assistance was experienced by 55 percent of the families.

This study considered individuals under age 65 as well as senior citizens. It also found that the families of younger patients are much more likely to experience severe financial burdens. This may be related to the lower household savings levels that exist for younger families. Also those over age 65 rarely suffer a loss of income when becoming seriously ill. The financial impact of these situations can be minimized by various supplemental financial protection insurance products, including cancer insurance, critical illness insurance, and hospital indemnity insurance.

13

■ Market Characteristics of the Purchaser

Various studies have shown that supplemental products are not bought by people of any specific demographic profile. Rather, they appeal to a cross-section of the population. In fact, people who purchase supplemental health insurance tend to fall into the broad middle range of Americans in terms of income, education, and occupation.

One study found virtually no differences between owners and nonowners of one supplemental product—hospital indemnity insurance—on any of the analytic variables. Researchers were struck with how similar the two groups of consumers seemed to be on a wide range of attitudes and behaviors: "People who think that long hospitalizations are common, people who are risk-averse, and people who are dependent on job income or who have few financial assets are all a little more likely than others to have purchased hospital indemnity insurance."[7(p.3)]

Perhaps more importantly, studies show that people purchase this coverage not instead of basic medical expense insurance, but in addition to it. In part this may be due to the fact that earlier basic medical policies had limited room-and-board benefits. A study by one large supplemental health insurance company showed that nearly 80 percent of its policyholders are covered under a primary health care plan such as comprehensive medical insurance, HMOs, or other managed care programs.[8] The study also showed market demographics for the company's supplemental products for income, education, and occupation.

Income

Three-quarters of the policyholders of supplemental health insurance have annual incomes between $10,000 and $49,000. Sixty-one percent of the U.S. population earns between these amounts. Therefore, these supplemental purchasers tend to be middle income individuals, with fewer people at the extreme lower and higher income levels. This could be because these coverages are not marketed to people eligible for Medicaid, and the higher income individuals may be more able to self-insure many of the supplemental risks.

Education

Seventy-seven percent of supplemental insurance purchasers are high school graduates or beyond, a percentage that corresponds almost exactly to the percentage of the U.S. population that holds high school diplomas and college and advanced degrees—78 percent in 1991. This is another indication that supplemental health insurance products have broad appeal and that supplemental purchasers resemble the whole population.

Occupation

One-third of supplemental policyholders are employed as managers, business owners, or professionals, which is slightly higher than the U.S. average. About half of the group (52 percent) are employed in blue-collar occupations (compared with the U.S. average of 43 percent), and perhaps of most interest, 54 percent work for firms of fewer than 25 employees. These firms typically are the ones that are unable to provide substantial employee benefit packages.

■ General Product Characteristics

Supplemental products have a number of unique characteristics that distinguish them from other plans (which can have complex underwriting, much larger premiums, multiple rate classes, rate increases, elimination periods, and coordination of benefits). One exception is Medicare supplement policies, which have rate increases. Characteristics of supplemental products are covered in this section.

Underwriting

Most supplemental accident and health insurance plans are offered with little or no underwriting, thus allowing the greatest number of people to qualify for coverage. This simplified approach is possible because of the generally objective nature of the benefit triggers involved with these products. For example, accident-only policies require that an accident

SUPPLEMENTAL HEALTH INSURANCE

must have occurred; hospital indemnity policies require hospital confinement. Such benefit triggers act to reduce the possibility of claimants manipulating their claim situations.

For some supplemental products, there are simplified underwriting requirements. The application may ask a limited number of health questions that directly relate to the coverage being provided. For example, a cancer policy application may ask about the applicant's history of cancer. Other policies reduce the impact of antiselection by excluding any pre-existing condition from coverage during the first 6 or 12 months the policy is in force. These alternative forms of underwriting help to minimize the expense of underwriting and speed the policy issue process.

The underwriting approaches for Medicare supplement plans are mandated by federal law. As people first become eligible for Medicare, they are guaranteed that any supplemental policy will be issued without any underwriting questions asked. Some contracts are issued covering all conditions while others exclude pre-existing conditions for a period of up to six months. After individuals have been enrolled in Medicare for six months, underwriting questions may be asked on any application for a new supplemental policy. However, if a Medicare supplement policy replaces an existing Medicare supplement policy, then the new policy must credit the time period that the original policy was in force toward any pre-existing condition exclusion period.

Pre-Existing Conditions

According to the National Association of Insurance Commissioners (NAIC), a pre-existing condition means the existence of symptoms that cause an ordinarily prudent person to seek diagnosis, care, or treatment within a five-year period preceding the effective date of the coverage of the insured person, or a condition for which medical advice or treatment was recommended by a physician or received from a physician within a five-year period preceding the effective date of the coverage of the insured person.

Insurance companies may vary their definition of pre-existing conditions by using time frames less (but never more) than the five years outlined in the NAIC model. Some companies provide coverage immediately for pre-existing conditions; others only consider pre-existing conditions during a 6-, 12-, or 24-month period prior to the effective date of the coverage.

Insurers also may vary the length of time they may require a policyholder to wait before their pre-existing condition is covered. Some companies provide immediate coverage; others require the insured to wait several months. Some pre-existing conditions are excluded completely from coverage.

Stable Premiums

The basic pricing of supplemental products is often constructed so that the price does not automatically change as the insured ages. In some cases, this is accomplished by charging the same rate for all ages. In others, the customer is charged a rate that varies only by the age of the insured at the time the premium is purchased. In these situations, it is anticipated that the insured would continue to pay the same rate for as long as the policy is in force. Rate increases only become necessary if the cost of benefits exceeds the pricing expectations held when the product was initially developed.

The benefits payable under many supplemental insurance policies are paid at a fixed rate on a daily or monthly basis. The benefits generally do not increase with inflation.

Even in supplemental products where benefits regularly increase, such as Medicare supplements, increases are usually in line with increases in Medicare deductibles and copayments and medical inflation.

Small Premium Size

Except for Medicare supplement premiums, which average close to $1,000 per person per year, annual rates for supplemental plans typically are less than $500, and in many cases less than $200. The small premiums of these products have many implications concerning how

17

the policies are administered. The administration must be very efficient in order to operate within the dollars available in the pricing margin. Premium billing and collection must be handled in a cost-effective way. Underwriting and claim functions must minimize the time and money spent qualifying the customer. Often, benefits are structured to assist in this process. Even when using simplified administrative approaches that reduce the cost, these expenses tend to be a higher proportion of the premium than they are for larger premium products.

Guaranteed Renewable or Noncancellable

Purchasers of supplemental coverage want the assurance that they will be able to continue their coverage in force regardless of changes in health. Guaranteed renewable contracts provide this type of assurance. Under these policies the prices can be raised on a class if the level of benefits exceeds pricing expectations. Medicare supplement policies, specified disease contracts, and most other supplemental products contain this type of renewal guarantee.

Some supplemental products are structured to be noncancellable. Under these products the company guarantees that the rate will not be changed and that the policy can be renewed for as long as the customer wants, until at least a certain age, such as 65. This is possible due to the stability of the underlying risk. This type of renewability often is found with accident-only coverages and sometimes with hospital indemnity coverages.

Broad Rate Classes

Supplemental coverages typically use simplified rating structures. For example, rates may not vary by age or by occupation class. If occupation class is used, the structure is highly simplified. For example, a supplemental plan may have one rate for all office employees and a different rate for all nonoffice employees. A traditional disability income policy would have four or five rate classes and a manual that defines the appropriate class for each possible occupation. Use of smoker-non-smoker rates is infrequent, and substandard rating is rare. A level premium structure based on age-at-issue is customary. These simplified rating structures facilitate administration and customer understanding.

Personally Owned

Supplemental plans are owned and paid for by the individual. The policy may be kept in force, regardless of change in employment or residence, at the personal discretion of the purchaser. Similarly, claim payments are made directly to the policyholder to be used for any purpose.

No Coordination of Benefits

Individual supplemental plans pay without regard to other coverage and do not coordinate benefits. This is an important characteristic of supplemental plans, and it enhances their appeal. Supplemental plans allow the consumer the ultimate choice of how he/she uses the benefits.

■ Overview of Supplemental Products

There are many types of products covering a wide variety of contingencies in today's supplemental health insurance marketplace. To appeal to specific consumer need, products often are designed for special situations or segments of the market. The following is a brief description of the supplemental products covered in greater detail in this book.

Medicare Supplement Insurance

The health insurance needs of people aged 65 and over are taken care of, to a great extent, by the federal Medicare program. However, because of Medicare's deductible, coinsurance, and limited benefits package, senior citizens are not fully protected against the considerable loss that may result from long-term hospitalization or prolonged medical

SUPPLEMENTAL HEALTH INSURANCE

expenses. Medicare supplement insurance helps pay some of these costs.

As of November 1991, all Medicare supplement policies were required to be standardized into 10 plans. All insurance companies marketing these plans must offer the core plan, and they may offer any or all of the other nine plans. All of the 10 standardized plans contain the same set of core benefits. Medicare beneficiaries also can receive these benefits by enrolling in managed care plans. The basic benefits fill the gaps of the Medicare program by providing:

- copayment for hospital charges from the 61st to the 90th day of hospital confinement;
- copayment for hospital charges associated with the insured's lifetime reserve bank for the 91st through 150th day of hospital confinement;
- entire cost of any excess (beyond 150 days) hospital confinement, up to 365 days;
- payment for blood transfusions; and
- Medicare Part B coinsurance.

In addition, the nine optional plans provide various combinations of the following benefits:

- daily copayments for treatment in a skilled nursing facility for the 21st day through the 100th day;
- Medicare Part A deductible;
- coverage for foreign travel;
- payment for services that allow at-home recovery;
- preventive medical care;
- prescription drugs; and
- Medicare Part B deductible.

Hospital Indemnity Insurance

Hospital indemnity coverage pays benefits for each day the insured is confined in a hospital. Benefits are paid for each day of covered hospital confinement, for either a sickness or injury. The maximum benefit period can range from 365 days up to life. Hospital indemnity benefits usually are paid without regard to any other benefits. The benefit normally is stated in a flat dollar amount per day. Indemnity amounts range from $30 to $400 per day. These products often provide higher amounts per day in the event of care in an intensive care or coronary care unit.

In addition, hospital indemnity products often provide a daily benefit for convalescence at home following hospitalization. The benefit for convalescence can be for an amount that is either the same as the in-hospital benefit or at a reduced level, such as 50 percent of the daily benefit. The payments may continue for a period linked to the duration of hospital confinement, such as one or two times the length of stay, or they may continue for a specified benefit period of disablement, such as for up to six months.

Specified Disease Insurance

The most common type of specified disease policy is cancer insurance. Many insurers offer one or more cancer policies to individuals and families to meet their needs for supplemental cancer protection.

Cancer insurance is purchased to fill the gaps in coverage for medical and/or related expenses (e.g., deductibles, coinsurance, and noncovered expenses). The benefits usually are paid without regard to any other type of medical insurance. Cancer insurance also provides protection against additional expenses such as food and lodging while traveling to another city for treatment, child care expense, and transportation costs often related to treating cancer patients.

Some cancer policies provide benefits much like a major medical policy and pay benefits for items such as cancer screening tests, daily room and board, physician visits, nursing, and drugs and medicines. Maximum benefits of $50,000 to $150,000 are common. These benefits usually are paid without regard to any other type of medical insurance.

Another type of specified disease insurance is critical illness coverage. These policies provide lump sum benefits upon the first diagnosis of one of several major illnesses or certain types of major surgery. Some policies require that the insured survive the diagnosis or the surgery for at least 30 days to be eligible for benefits. This requirement highlights the fact that the products are designed to assist the insured during his or her recovery rather than being a limited form of life insurance. The illnesses usually include cancer, heart attack, and stroke. In addition, other critical conditions may be included, such as kidney failure, major organ replacement, heart surgery, brain tumor, multiple sclerosis, paralysis or dismemberment, severe burns, or blindness.

Critical illness coverage is becoming more popular because it is believed that more people are surviving these episodes than has previously been the case and that more care is needed for the patient's recovery. Although the benefit received is usually 100 percent of the lump sum selected, for some conditions lower percentages are applicable.

Accident Insurance

There are several kinds of accident policies designed to cover specific needs.

Accident Medical Expense Insurance

Accident medical expense coverage generally applies only if the expenses are incurred within a specified time (usually three or six months) from the date of the accident. Benefits are subject to an overall maximum benefit for any one accident. Some insurers offer individual accident medical plans that exceed these benefit levels. Some plans have small deductibles (e.g., $25); others provide first-dollar coverage.

The benefits, whether group or individual, cover necessary treatment following an accidental injury. Typically the following benefits are included:

- treatment by a physician;
- hospital care;
- registered nursing (RN) care; and
- X-ray and laboratory examinations.

Accident Hospital Indemnity Policies

Accident hospital indemnity policies are similar to hospital indemnity policies except that benefits are payable only in the event of hospitalization due to a covered accident. The amount paid for each day of confinement is specifically stated in the policy. In some policies the daily confinement benefit increases each year that the policy is in force. Additional benefits payable for other accident-related contingencies are often included in these policies, such as daily benefits for intensive care or post-hospitalization convalescence, benefits for emergency room treatment, death, dismemberment, disability, or medical treatment.

Accidental Death and Dismemberment Insurance (AD&D)

AD&D benefits are payable when an insured person dies or loses the sight of one or both eyes, or loses one hand or a foot directly as a result of an accidental bodily injury. In some products, the insured needs to only loose the use of hand or foot in order to collect benefits. Actual dismemberment is not required. This coverage may be written as 24-hour or as nonoccupational insurance. Twenty-four-hour insurance provides benefits at any time for an accident incurred either on or off the job. Nonoccupational insurance does not provide benefits for an accident arising out of the insured's employment.

Accident Disability

Accident disability benefits, which provide monthly income to the insured, are payable only when the cause of disability is due to an accident. As with AD&D, accident disability insurance is sold either as 24-hour coverage or nonoccupational coverage.

Travel Accident

Travel accident insurance covers motor vehicle accidents and accidents on scheduled airlines and other common carriers, including taxis, buses, and subways. Coverage can be for one trip, a specific period, or continuous. Benefits are payable only if the insured is in an accident that occurred during the covered trip. Payment is usually a lump sum up to about

$1 million for scheduled airline benefits. Some plans add daily hospitalization benefits for accidental injuries incurred during the covered trip.

Dental Insurance

Dental benefits provide reimbursement for the expenses of dental services and supplies, including preventive care. The major classifications of dental services include:

- diagnostic;
- preventive;
- restorative (including fillings, inlays, and crowns);
- prosthodontics (installment and maintenance of bridgework);
- oral surgery;
- periodontics or endodontics (treatment of gums); and
- orthodontics (straightening treatment).

Benefits may be provided through a plan integrated with medical expense insurance coverages, or a plan may be written separately from other coverages (nonintegrated or stand-alone).

Integrated Plans

Dental expenses under an integrated plan are blended into the covered expenses of a major medical benefits plan. Generally, coverage is on a usual and customary or nonscheduled basis. The deductible must be satisfied each calendar year by medical expenses, dental care expenses, or both. The amount payable for dental and medical care expenses usually is subject to the same coinsurance percentage. Sometimes dental care expenses are separated into classes or categories of services (restorative, prosthodontics, orthodontics, and so forth), and a different coinsurance level is applied to each class.

Nonintegrated Plans

Dental expenses under a nonintegrated plan are covered separately on either a scheduled or nonscheduled basis. A schedule of dental services, similar to a surgical schedule, lists specific procedures. Reimbursement toward the dentist's charges is up to the amount specified in the schedule for each procedure. Nonscheduled dental plans provide reimbursement toward the dentist's charges for all covered dental services on a usual and customary basis, similar to an integrated plan.

Specialty Plans

There are several specialty supplemental plans on the market today. This book discusses three of them: prescription drugs, vision, and TRICARE supplement. Examples of other specialty plans are programs that provide for emergency medical treatment for people traveling abroad; medical treatment for participants in athletic events; or rescue and medical treatment for hikers, skiers, or mountain climbers.

Prescription Drug Insurance

Prescription drug insurance covers drugs and medicines purchased on the order of a physician. Most plans are offered through an employer on a group basis at very little or no cost to the insured. There are two basic plans: reimbursement and service.

Reimbursement plans. Reimbursement plans require the individual to pay for the prescription drugs and to submit these expenses to the insurer on a claim form completed by the pharmacist or the insured. Payment is made to the individual based on the insurer's determination of usual and customary charges.

Service plans. Service plans refer to a system in which payment by the insurer is made directly to the provider for the service or product covered by the insurance policy without the insured having to file a claim. Mail-order prescription drug plans provide a 60- or 90-day supply of drugs and require the insured to make a copayment, which typically ranges from $5 to $15. The insurer pays the provider the rest.

Vision Care Insurance

Vision care insurance is designed to provide benefits for routine preventive and corrective eye care. It usually is written to complement other basic group coverages. The primary objective is to encourage regular or periodic eye examinations so that appropriate corrective measures may be taken. Under most vision care programs, the services covered require the authorization of an ophthalmologist or optometrist.

Vision care benefits provide reimbursement for:

- eye examinations (including refraction);
- single vision, bifocal, and trifocal lenses;
- contact lenses;
- other aids for subnormal vision; and
- frames (limitation on the dollar amount, due to the variable cost of these items).

Vision plans reimburse insureds in one of three ways:

- a flat dollar amount per individual (e.g., $150) toward all covered services provided in a calendar year;
- coverage on a usual and customary basis; or
- coverage based on a specified schedule.

TRICARE Supplement

TRICARE is the health insurance program for members of the Uniformed Services and their families in the civilian community. As the replacement for the Civilian Health and Medical Program of the Uniformed Services (CHAMPUS) in 1997, TRICARE covers spouses and dependents of active duty personnel, reservists, and retirees who are affiliated with the Army, Navy, Marine Corps, Air Force, Coast Guard, Public Health Service, and National Oceanic and Atmospheric Administration. Eligibility for TRICARE ends at age 65, when covered people become eligible for Medicare.

TRICARE supplement products generally cover some part of the deductibles, coinsurance, and cost share amounts associated with the TRICARE program.

■ Summary

Supplemental health policies play an important role in the insurance marketplace by filling the gaps left by basic, primary health care insurance. They allow the expansion of coverage beyond the benefits provided by an employer and help people preserve their standard of living in the unfortunate event of a financially challenging injury or illness.

The wide variety of supplemental products available is to be expected, as there is a wide variety of insurance needs that people want to protect. Some products focus on covering medical expenses; others focus on covering related expenses, and some replace lost income. Consumers can customize their total insurance packets to fit their special needs and concerns.

The products are purchased by a broad cross-section of the population. Typically, they contain features that are easily understood, benefits are predictable, and rates tend to be stable. Generally, customer satisfaction is quite high. These factors have enhanced the acceptance of supplemental products and encouraged the expansion of the supplemental health insurance market.

■ Key Terms

Accident hospital indemnity insurance
Accident medical expense insurance
Accidental death and dismemberment (AD&D) insurance
Dental insurance
First-day coverage
Guaranteed renewable
Health care coverages
Hospital indemnity insurance
Medical expenses
Medicare supplement insurance
Noncancellable
Premiums
Prescription drug insurance
Rate classes
Related expenses
Specified disease insurance
Supplemental health insurance
TRICARE supplement
Underwriting
Vision insurance

Chapter 2

MEDICARE SUPPLEMENTS

29 *Introduction*
31 *Customer Needs*
39 *Benefits*
51 *Underwriting*

52 *Rating*
55 *Regulations*
60 *Summary*
61 *Key Terms*

∎ Introduction

More than 38 million older and disabled Americans get health care coverage under Medicare, the federal health insurance program created in 1965 by amendments to the Social Security Act (Health Insurance for the Aged Act—Title XVIII). Prior to Medicare, only 50 percent of the elderly population had any type of health insurance. Now, only 1 percent of the elderly are uninsured.[9] The Medicare program paid a total of $176.9 billion dollars on behalf of beneficiaries in 1995 (an average of $4,660 per enrollee). This figure is expected to reach $295 billion by the year 2000.[10] With a larger population and longer life expectancies, Medicare enrollment will continue to climb.

To understand the need for Medicare supplements, it is necessary to understand the federal Medicare program. Medicare encompasses two health care programs: a hospital benefit plan (Part A) and a medical plan (Part B). The health insurance needs of people aged 65 and older, certain younger disabled people, and people with permanent kidney failure should be taken care of by the Medicare program. However, because of deductible and coinsurance requirements and limits on Medicare allowable charges, persons covered under Medicare are not fully protected against the considerable losses that may result from long-term hospitalization or prolonged and costly medical expenses. Medicare supplements (often referred to as Medigap or MedSup policies) are designed to fill the benefit gaps in the Medicare program.

SUPPLEMENTAL HEALTH INSURANCE

Medicare is run by the Health Care Financing Administration (HCFA) of the U.S. Department of Health and Human Services. The Social Security Administration assists HCFA by enrolling eligible people into the Medicare program and collecting Medicare premiums.

Part A of Medicare is financed by part of the social security payroll withholding tax paid by workers and their employers and by part of the self-employment tax paid by self-employed persons. Generally, there is no monthly premium at age 65 if a person has worked for at least 10 years in Medicare-covered employment. This includes workers who have had their social security taxes paid either through their employer or, if self-employed, through their self-employment tax. Individuals who do not qualify for premium-free Part A may buy it if they are at least 65 years old and meet certain requirements. The monthly premium is based on the amount of covered quarters of Medicare-covered employment.

Part B is a voluntary program. Eligible persons automatically are enrolled in the program when they become entitled to premium-free Part A, unless they state that they do not want it. Twenty-five percent of Part B costs are paid by the participant in premiums; the balance is paid by the federal government. Part B premiums are deducted from participants' social security, railroad retirement, or civil service retirement checks. Part B also may be purchased if a person does not qualify for premium-free Part A.

The Balanced Budget Act of 1997 established a new Part C—Medicare +Choice. Enrollees of Medicare+Choice pay the Part B premium. As an alternative to electing the existing package of Medicare benefits through the traditional Medicare fee-for-service program, every individual entitled to Medicare Part A and enrolled in Part B will be able to choose from the following plans:

- private fee-for-service plans;
- preferred provider organizations;
- health maintenance organizations (HMOs), some with point-of-service (POS) features;
- provider-sponsored organizations (PSOs);

- medical savings account (MSA) and high deductible plan, a demonstration program limited to 390,000 beneficiaries; and
- private fee-for-service opt-out (no Medicare or Medicare+Choice reimbursement).

■ Customer Needs

Gaps in Coverage

Because Medicare was designed with deductibles and coinsurance and with limits on covered services, there have been gaps in coverage from the beginning. Table 2.1 shows the deductible and coinsurance amounts from 1966, the first year of the Medicare program, until 1998. Part A deductibles and coinsurance amounts have increased every year since 1969; Part B deductibles have doubled during the same period.

As these deductibles and coinsurance amounts increase, so does the need for a Medicare supplement policy, which pays the benefits not paid for by Medicare. On average, Medicare covers only about 45 percent of the health expenditures of people aged 65 and older (70 percent of hospital bills, 61 percent of physicians' charges, and 15 percent of other personal health care services).[11] Beneficiary satisfaction with the combined coverage of Medicare and Medicare supplements is extremely high compared with beneficiary satisfaction with Medicare coverage alone. (See Figure 2.1.)

Part A (Hospitalization)

Medicare hospital and skilled nursing facility benefits (Part A) are paid on the basis of benefit periods. A benefit period begins the first day a person receives a Medicare-covered service as an inpatient in a qualified hospital and ends when the person has been out of a hospital or other facility that mainly provides skilled nursing or rehabilitation services for 60 days in a row. Should a person go back to a qualified hospital after 60 days, a new benefit period begins, the hospital and skilled nursing facility benefits are renewed and the initial hospital deductible must be

SUPPLEMENTAL HEALTH INSURANCE

Table 2.1
History of Medicare Components

Year	Part A inpatient hospital deductible	Part A inpatient hospital coinsurance 61–90 days	Part A inpatient hospital coinsurance 91–150 days (lifetime reserve)	Part A coinsurance skilled nursing facility 21–100 days	% Change	Annual Part B deductible	% Change	Part B premium	% Change
1966	40.00	10.00	N/A	N/A	N/A	50.00	N/A	3.00	N/A
1967	40.00	10.00	N/A	5.00	0.0	50.00	0.0	3.00	0.0
1968	40.00	10.00	20.00	5.00	0.0	50.00	0.0	4.00	33.3
1969	44.00	11.00	22.00	5.50	10.0	50.00	0.0	4.00	0.0
1970	52.00	13.00	26.00	6.50	18.2	50.00	0.0	5.30	32.5
1971	60.00	15.00	30.00	7.50	15.4	50.00	0.0	5.60	5.7
1972	68.00	17.00	34.00	8.50	13.3	50.00	0.0	5.80	3.6
1973	72.00	18.00	36.00	9.00	5.9	60.00	20.0	6.30	8.6
1974	84.00	21.00	42.00	10.50	16.7	60.00	0.0	6.70	6.4
1975	92.00	23.00	46.00	11.50	9.5	60.00	0.0	6.70	0.0
1976	104.00	26.00	52.00	13.00	13.0	60.00	0.0	7.20	7.7
1977	124.00	31.00	62.00	15.50	19.2	60.00	0.0	7.70	6.9
1978	144.00	36.00	72.00	18.00	16.1	60.00	0.0	8.20	6.5
1979	160.00	40.00	80.00	20.00	11.1	60.00	0.0	8.70	6.1
1980	180.00	45.00	90.00	22.50	12.5	60.00	0.0	9.60	10.3
1981	204.00	51.00	102.00	25.50	13.3	60.00	0.0	11.00	14.6
1982	260.00	65.00	130.00	32.50	27.5	75.00	25.0	12.20	10.9
1983	304.00	76.00	152.00	38.00	16.9	75.00	0.0	12.20	0.0
1984	356.00	89.00	178.00	44.50	17.1	75.00	0.0	14.60	19.7
1985	400.00	100.00	200.00	50.00	12.4	75.00	0.0	15.50	6.2
1986	492.00	123.00	246.00	61.50	23.0	75.00	0.0	15.50	0.0
1987	520.00	130.00	260.00	65.00	5.7	75.00	0.0	17.90	15.5
1988	540.00	135.00	270.00	67.50	3.8	75.00	0.0	24.80	38.5
1989	560.00	*	*	*	N/A	75.00	0.0	27.90	12.5
1990	592.00	148.00	296.00	74.00	N/A	75.00	0.0	28.60	2.5
1991	628.00	157.00	314.00	78.50	6.1	100.00	33.3	29.90	4.5
1992	652.00	163.00	326.00	81.50	3.8	100.00	0.0	31.80	6.3
1993	676.00	169.00	338.00	84.50	3.7	100.00	0.0	36.60	15.1
1994	696.00	174.00	348.00	87.00	2.9	100.00	0.0	41.10	12.3
1995	716.00	179.00	358.00	89.50	2.9	100.00	0.0	46.10	12.2
1996	736.00	184.00	368.00	92.00	2.8	100.00	0.0	42.50	(7.8)
1997	760.00	190.00	380.00	95.00	3.3	100.00	0.0	43.80	3.1
1998	764.00	191.00	382.00	95.50	0.005	100.00	0.0	43.80	0.0
1999									
2000									

*None due to passage by Congress of the Medicare Catastrophic Coverage Act of 1988. Act was repealed by Congress in 1989.
NOTE: N/A = Not Applicable

MEDICARE SUPPLEMENTS

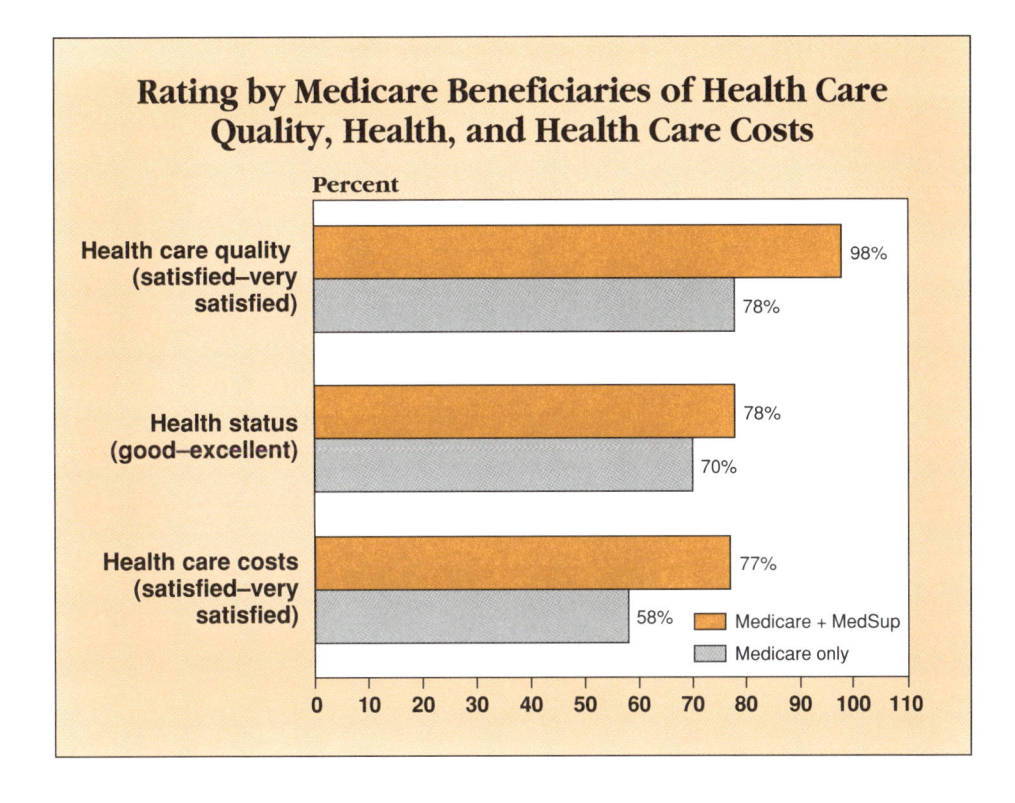

Rating by Medicare Beneficiaries of Health Care Quality, Health, and Health Care Costs

Percent

Health care quality (satisfied–very satisfied): Medicare + MedSup 98%, Medicare only 78%

Health status (good–excellent): Medicare + MedSup 78%, Medicare only 70%

Health care costs (satisfied–very satisfied): Medicare + MedSup 77%, Medicare only 58%

Figure 2.1

SOURCE: Khandker, R.K. and McCormack, L.A. Enrollment and Utilization Across Medicare Supplemental Plans, 1996. Center for Health Economics Research, Final Report to Health Care Financing Administration.

paid. There is no limit to the number of benefit periods a person may have for Part A benefits.

Part B (Medical)

Medical benefits (Part B) are paid based on a calendar year (January 1 through December 31). Each calendar year a person must pay a deductible ($100 in 1998). Then Medicare provides coverage for 80 percent of the Medicare-approved amount for all covered services received during the rest of the calendar year. The Medicare beneficiary is responsible for the remaining 20 percent of approved charges and noncovered charges.

Table 2.2 and Table 2.3 outline the services provided for by the Medicare program, the amount Medicare will pay for each service, and the amount each person must pay out of his/her own pocket when confronted with a hospital or medical bill.

Noncovered Charges

The following items are *not* covered under Medicare:

- acupuncture;
- most chiropractic services;
- cosmetic surgery (except after an accident);
- custodial care;
- dental care;
- most prescription drugs and medicines taken at home;
- eyeglasses and eye exams for prescribing, fitting, or changing glasses;
- routine foot care;
- most Canadian and Mexican health care;
- hearing aids and hearing examinations for prescribing, fitting, or changing hearing aids;
- homemaker services;
- immunizations (except vaccinations for pneumonia, hepatitis B, or influenza virus and immunizations due to an injury or immediate risk of infection);
- self-administered injections;
- meals delivered at home;
- naturopathic services;
- nursing care on a full-time basis in the home;
- orthopedic shoes (except as part of a leg brace);
- personal convenience items (e.g., phone, radio, or television in the hospital or skilled nursing facility);
- routine physical examinations and tests;
- private duty nurses;

MEDICARE SUPPLEMENTS

Table 2.2

Medicare (Part A) Hospital Services—Per Benefit Period

Services	Medicare pays	You pay
Hospitalization Semi-private room and board, general nursing services, and miscellaneous services and supplies		
First 60 days	All but $764.00 (Part A deductible)	$764
61st through 90th day	All but $191 a day	$191 a day
91st through 150th day (while using "lifetime reserve" days)	$382 a day	$382 a day
Beyond 150 days	Nothing	All costs
Skilled nursing facility care You must meet Medicare's requirements, including having been in a hospital for at least 3 days and entered a Medicare-approved facility within 30 days after leaving the hospital		
First 20 days	100% of approved amount	Nothing
Additional 80 days	All but $95.50 a day	Up to $95.50 a day
Beyond 100 days	Nothing	All costs
Hospice care Available as long as your physician certifies you are terminally ill and you elect to receive these services	All but limited costs for outpatient drugs and inpatient respite care	Limited cost sharing for outpatient drugs and inpatient respite care
Blood		
First 3 pints	Nothing	For first 3 pints
Additional amounts	All costs	Nothing

NOTE: A benefit period begins on the first day you receive service as an inpatient in a hospital and ends after you have been out of the hospital and have nor received skilled care in any other facility for 60 days in a row.

35

SUPPLEMENTAL HEALTH INSURANCE

Table 2.3

Medicare (Part B) Medical Services—Per Calendar Year

Services	Medicare pays	You pay
Medical expenses Such as physicians' services, inpatient and outpatient medical and surgical services and supplies, physical and speech therapy, diagnostic tests, durable medical equipment		
First $100 of Medicare-approved amount	Nothing (Part B deductible)	$100
Remainder of Medicare-approved amount	Generally 80%	Generally 20%
Part B excess charges (above Medicare-approved amount)	Nothing	All costs
Blood		
First 3 pints	Nothing	All costs
Additional amounts	80% of Medicare-approved amount (after $100 deductible)	20% of Medicare-approved amount (after $100 deductible)
Clinical laboratory services Blood test, urinalysis, and more	Generally 100% of approved amount	Nothing

NOTE: Once you have been billed $100 of Medicare-approved amounts for covered services, your Part B deductible will be met for the calendar year.

Medicare Parts A and B

Services	Medicare pays	You pay
Home health care Part-time or intermittent skilled care, home health aide services, and other services and supplies	100% of approved amount for services	Nothing
Durable medical equipment		
First $100 of Medicare-approved amount	Nothing	$100 (Part B deductible)
Remainder of approved amount	80% of Medicare-approved amount	20% of Medicare-approved amount

- private rooms;

- services rendered by a relative or member of the person's household;

- services payable by any of the following: workers' compensation, liability or no-fault insurance, employer group health plans for employees and their spouses, employer group health plans for people entitled to Medicare solely on the basis of end-stage renal disease, or another government program; and

- services for which there is no obligation to pay.

Distribution Methods

Medicare supplement plans have been on the market since the beginning of the Medicare program. Today, more than 29 million people are covered by a Medicare supplement policy. These policies are sold or provided through a variety of distribution channels including agents and brokers, employers, associations, and mass marketing. Of the 82 percent of people over age 65 who have supplemental coverage, 39 percent purchased a private Medicare supplement plan; 36 percent have supplemental coverage provided by their current or prior employer; and another 7 percent have both.[12]

Agents/Brokers

An insurance agent may represent one company (often referred to as a captive agent) or a number of different companies. The agent must be licensed by the state to sell and service Medicare supplement insurance to the public.

Agents who place Medicare supplement business with more than one company and who represent the insured rather than the insurance company are called brokers. The broker must also be licensed by the state where the policies are being sold. Both the agent and the broker receive a commission for the sale of each Medicare supplement policy.

Associations

When an applicant is a member of a professional or trade association, he/she may be eligible for group Medicare supplement insurance. Association insurance covers all members of the group under one master policy. Each member receives a certificate of insurance rather than an individual insurance policy. The association also may submit the premium to the insurance company for each member.

While association coverage must comply with the same federal and state regulations as individual Medicare supplement plans, association group products are required to meet a 75 percent lifetime loss ratio in contrast to a 65 percent lifetime loss ratio for individual products.

Employers

Employers may offer to help pay their retirees' Medicare supplement premiums or pay the entire premium as part of their overall health insurance program. The plans may be sold on an individual or group basis.

Mass Marketing

Many companies offer Medicare supplements to eligible people through the mail. People often choose this type of solicitation because they want to make the decision to buy on their own, without the involvement of an agent or broker. Companies in this market send out thousands of pieces of mail each year to individuals turning age 65. It is estimated that 5,000 people turn 65 every day, and by the year 2050 the Medicare-eligible population will have grown from the 38 million today to over 69 million.

Customer Service

Providing the highest quality customer service is an important part of most companies' strategic objectives. With companies offering standardized products, service is a critical component in the buying decision. People expect, many even demand, the best customer service each and every time they contact their insurance company. Companies that do not provide the highest degree of service may find their Medicare supplement business replaced by one of their competitors.

Many companies try to add value to their Medicare supplement business. This added-value benefit may take many forms. Electronic claims, for example, are faster and easier than traditional paper processing and provide a hassle-free, no paperwork process for the insured's claims.

■ Benefits

There are 10 standardized Medicare supplement plans (Plans A through J) that contain basic benefits and other benefits designed to fill the benefit gaps in the Medicare program. Table 2.4 shows the standard benefits of each plan and the sales distribution by plan. All Medicare supplements are required to automatically increase their benefits to adjust to Medicare's changes in deductible and coinsurance amounts. In addition, Medicare supplements are guaranteed renewable, which means that an insurance company may not cancel a policy for any reason except nonpayment of premiums. Premiums, however, can be revised on a class basis.

Plan A

Plan A is often referred to as the core plan, since the basic benefit structure of Plan A is included in the other nine Medicare supplement policies. The basic benefits of Plan A provide the following coverage:

- Part A coinsurance amount from the 61st day through the 90th day of hospitalization in each Medicare benefit period;
- Part A coinsurance amount from the 91st day through the 150th day (these days represent the 60 nonrenewable lifetime hospital reserve days);
- after 150 days, when Medicare's benefits have run out, 100 percent of Medicare Part A–eligible hospital expenses (limited to a maximum of 365 days of additional inpatient hospital days during the insured's lifetime);

SUPPLEMENTAL HEALTH INSURANCE

Table 2.4

Ten Standard Medicare Supplement Plans and Sales Distribution

Basic benefits included in all plans:
Hospitalization: Part A coinsurance plus coverage for 385 additional days after Medicare benefits end.
Medical Expenses: Part B coinsurance (generally 20% of Medicare-approved expenses).
Blood: First 3 pints each year.

A	B	C	D	E	F	G	H	I	J
Basic benefit	Basic benefit	Basic benefit	Basic benefit	Basic benefit	Basic benefit	Basic benefit	Basic benefit	Basic benefit	Basic benefit
	Part A deductible	Part A deductible	Skilled nursing coinsurance	Skilled nursing coinsurance	Skilled nursing coinsurance	Skilled nursing coinsurance	Skilled nursing coinsurance	Skilled nursing coinsurance	Skilled nursing coinsurance
		Part B deductible	Part A deductible	Part A deductible	Part A deductible	Part A deductible	Part A deductible	Part A deductible	Part A deductible
					Part B deductible				Part B deductible
					Part B excess (100%)	Part B excess (80%)		Part B excess (100%)	Part B excess (100%)
		Foreign travel emergency	Foreign travel emergency	Foreign travel emergency	Foreign travel emergency	Foreign travel emergency	Foreign travel emergency	Foreign travel emergency	Foreign travel emergency
			At-home recovery			At-home recovery		At-home recovery	At-home recovery
							Basic drug benefit ($1,250 limit)	Basic drug benefit ($1,250 limit)	Basic drug benefit ($3,000 limit)
				Preventive care					Preventive care

Distribution of Sales (1992–1993)

| 7.0% | 16.3% | 22.0% | 4.4% | 1.2% | 32.7% | 2.3% | 6.0% | 3.3% | 4.8% |

SOURCE: Health Care Financing Administration. *1997 Guide to Health Insurance for People with Medicare*. Sales distribution from a 1992-1993 survey of insurance carriers cited in the 1996 Annual Report to Congress of the Physician Payment Review Commission.

- reasonable cost of the first three pints of blood under parts A and B; and

- Part B coinsurance amount (generally 20 percent of the approved amount or 50 percent of the approved charges for outpatient mental health services) after the calendar year deductible of $100.

Plan B

Plan B contains all of the basic benefits of the core plan, *plus* the following coverage:

- Part A inpatient hospital deductible.

Plan C

Plan C contains all of the basic benefits of the core plan, *plus* the following coverage:

- Part A inpatient hospital deductible;
- skilled nursing facility care coinsurance amount from days 21 through 100, per benefit period;
- Part B calendar year deductible ($100); and
- 80 percent of the medically necessary emergency care received in a foreign country, after a $250 deductible, up to a lifetime maximum of $50,000.

Plan D

Plan D contains all of the basic benefits of the core plan, *plus* the following coverage:

- Part A inpatient hospital deductible;
- skilled nursing facility care coinsurance amount from days 21 through 100, per benefit period;

SUPPLEMENTAL HEALTH INSURANCE

- 80 percent of the medically necessary emergency care received in a foreign country, after a $250 deductible, up to a lifetime maximum of $50,000; and

- up to $1,600 per year for short-term, at-home assistance with activities of daily living (e.g., bathing, dressing, personal hygiene) when recovering from an illness, injury, or surgery.

Plan E

Plan E contains all of the basic benefits of the core plan, *plus* the following coverage:

- Part A inpatient hospital deductible;
- skilled nursing facility care coinsurance amount from days 21 through 100, per benefit period;
- 80 percent of the medically necessary emergency care received in a foreign country, after a $250 deductible, up to a lifetime maximum of $50,000; and
- up to $120 per year for physicals, cholesterol screenings, hearing tests, diabetes screenings, and thyroid function tests.

Plan F

Plan F contains all of the basic benefits of the core plan, *plus* the following coverage:

- Part A inpatient hospital deductible;
- skilled nursing facility care coinsurance amount from days 21 through 100, per benefit period;
- Part B calendar year deductible ($100);
- 80 percent of the medically necessary emergency care received in a foreign country, after a $250 deductible, up to a lifetime maximum of $50,000; and
- 100 percent of the Part B excess charges. This coverage pays the difference between the actual Medicare Part B charge as billed and the

Medicare-approved charge, not to exceed the charge limitation established by Medicare (115 percent of the Medicare-approved amount). Only physicians who do not accept Medicare assignment may bill their patients for charges above the Medicare-approved amount. For example, if the Medicare-approved amount for a particular service is $100, then the physician who does not accept assignment may bill his/her patient up to $115 for that service; this plan will reimburse up to $15.

Plan G

Plan G contains all of the basic benefits of the core plan, *plus* the following coverage:

- Part A inpatient hospital deductible;
- skilled nursing facility care coinsurance amount from days 21 through 100, per benefit period;
- 80 percent of the Part B excess charges. This coverage pays the difference between the actual Medicare Part B charge as billed and the Medicare-approved charge, not to exceed the charge limitation established by Medicare (115 percent of the Medicare approved amount);
- 80 percent of the medically necessary emergency care received in a foreign country, after a $250 deductible up to a lifetime maximum of $50,000; and
- up to $1,600 per year for short-term, at-home assistance with activities of daily living (e.g., bathing, dressing, personal hygiene) when recovering from an illness, injury, or surgery.

Plan H

Plan H contains all of the basic benefits of the core plan, *plus* the following coverage:

- Part A inpatient hospital deductible;
- skilled nursing facility care coinsurance amount from days 21 through 100, per benefit period;

SUPPLEMENTAL HEALTH INSURANCE

- 80 percent of the medically necessary emergency care received in a foreign country, after a $250 deductible, up to a lifetime maximum of $50,000; and

- 50 percent of the cost of prescription drugs up to a maximum benefit of $1,250, after a calendar year deductible of $250. This prescription drug benefit is referred to as the basic drug benefit.

Plan I

Plan I contains all of the basic benefits of the core plan, *plus* the following coverage:

- Part A inpatient hospital deductible;

- skilled nursing facility care coinsurance amount from days 21 through 100, per benefit period;

- 100 percent of the Part B excess charges. This coverage pays the difference between the actual Medicare Part B charge as billed and the Medicare-approved charge, not to exceed the charge limitation established by Medicare (115 percent of the Medicare-approved amount);

- 80 percent of the medically necessary emergency care received in a foreign country, after a $250 deductible, up to a lifetime maximum of $50,000;

- Up to $1,600 per year for short-term, at-home assistance with activities of daily living (e.g., bathing, dressing, personal hygiene) when recovering from an illness, injury, or surgery; and

- 50 percent of the cost of prescription drugs up to a maximum benefit of $1,250, after a calendar year deductible of $250. This prescription drug benefit is referred to as the basic drug benefit.

Plan J

Plan J contains a combination of all of the benefits available under the other Medicare supplement plans. It is the most comprehensive Medicare supplement product a person may buy. Plan J contains all of the basic benefits of the core plan, *plus* the following coverage:

- Part A inpatient hospital deductible;
- skilled nursing facility care coinsurance amount from days 21 through 100, per benefit period;
- Part B calendar year deductible ($100);
- 100 percent of the Part B excess charges. This coverage pays the difference between the actual Medicare Part B charge as billed and the Medicare-approved charge, not to exceed the charge limitation established by Medicare (115 percent of the Medicare-approved amount);
- 80 percent of the medically necessary emergency care received in a foreign country, after a $250 deductible up to a lifetime maximum of $50,000;
- up to $120 per year for physicals, cholesterol screenings, hearing tests, diabetes screenings, and thyroid function tests;
- up to $1,600 per year for short-term, at-home assistance with activities of daily living (e.g., bathing, dressing, personal hygiene) when recovering from an illness, injury, or surgery.
- 50 percent of the cost of prescription drugs up to a maximum benefit of $3,000, after a calendar year deductible of $250. This prescription drug benefit is referred to as the extended drug benefit.

Exceptions and Limitations

All Medicare supplements have exceptions and limitations in their contracts. In addition, they do not provide benefits for services not covered under Medicare, unless specifically provided for in the contract. For example, Medicare does not provide benefits for prescription drugs, but prescription drugs are covered up to the plan's limit under Plans H, I, and J. Medicare supplements may not be issued with a benefit limitation (e.g., 12-month wait) or disease elimination (e.g., no coverage for a specific health condition).

Insurers are permitted to limit or exclude coverage for services related to a pre-existing health condition when a Medicare supplement policy is sold (whether or not during an open enrollment period). Such a limitation, however, cannot be imposed for a period of more than six months. Certain continuously enrolled individuals are guaranteed the

SUPPLEMENTAL HEALTH INSURANCE

issuance of a Medicare supplement policy without a pre-existing condition limitation. The law prohibits an insurer from discriminating in the pricing of such policy on the basis of the individual's health status, claims experience, receipt of health care, or medical condition.

When making a decision to buy a Medicare supplement policy, a person should know what types of services and supplies are not covered by Medicare and, therefore, are not generally covered by a Medicare supplement policy.

Medicare SELECT

Insurance companies and health maintenance organizations (HMOs) sell another type of Medicare supplement referred to as a Medicare SELECT plan. Medicare SELECT is the same as standard Medicare supplement coverage except that each insurer has specific hospitals and physicians that must be used (except in an emergency situation) for full Medicare SELECT benefits to be payable. Medicare SELECT plans generally are less expensive because of the requirement to use only network providers to obtain full benefits. The Medicare SELECT program offers more flexibility than an HMO concerning a patient's choice of physicians because insureds can go to physicians outside the network and still receive partial benefits; this is not allowed in an HMO.

Insurers who offer Medicare SELECT plans are required to file a proposed plan of operation with the commissioner of insurance of the state where they wish to sell their Medicare SELECT plan. The plan must include:

- evidence that all covered services that are subject to restricted network provisions are available and accessible through network providers, including a demonstration that (1) services are provided with reasonable promptness, with respect to geographic location, hours of operation, and after-hours care; (2) the number of providers in the area are sufficient for the number of expected policy owners; (3) a written agreement with each provider describes the plan's responsibilities; (4) emergency care is available 24 hours a day, 7 days a week; and (5) providers may not seek direct reimbursement from an individual covered under the Medicare SELECT plan;

- a statement or map providing a clear description of the service area;
- a description of the grievance procedure to be used;
- a description of the quality assurance program, including (1) formal organizational structure; (2) written criteria for selection, retention, and removal of network providers; and (3) procedures for evaluating the quality of care provided by network providers and the process to initiate corrective action when needed;
- a list and description, by specialty, of the network providers;
- copies of all written information that the insurer proposes to use; and
- any other information requested by the insurance commissioner.

Congress designed Medicare SELECT as an experimental program and initially approved the program as part of the Omnibus Reconciliation Act of 1990 (OBRA-90) for use in 15 states. It was later approved by Congress for all 50 states and extended until the end of 1998. Carriers must provide coverage if SELECT plans are discontinued. The insurer must provide benefits that are similar to the benefits contained in the Medicare SELECT plan.

Although the Medicare SELECT program is potentially available in every state under federal law, not all states have approved these plans for sale. This information should be available by calling the insurance department in a particular state.

Medicare and HMOs

As an alternative to Plans A through J, whether regular or Medicare SELECT, beneficiaries can enroll in a risk plan that includes all of the benefits of Medicare and generally a number of supplemental benefits, such as eye exams, hearing aids, routine physicals, and scheduled immunizations for little or no extra premium. Individuals must continue to pay their Part B premium to Medicare. Medicare's deductible and coinsurance amounts are paid by the HMO, not the insured. HMOs also require little or no paperwork.

Enrollment in HMOs is increasing rapidly. In 1995, 3.3 million Medicare enrollees chose HMOs—a 23 percent increase between 1994 and 1995.

By 2000, 11.8 million Medicare enrollees are expected to be enrolled in HMOs. The number of HMOs that have contracts with HCFA also is increasing. In 1995, almost one-third of all commercial HMOs (168 plans) held contracts to serve Medicare beneficiaries. Seventy-one percent of enrollment in these plans is concentrated in six states: California, Florida, Minnesota, New York, Oregon, and Texas.[13]

Generally, a Medicare risk plan must have its own network of hospitals, skilled nursing facilities, home health agencies, physicians, and other professionals. Depending on how the plan is organized, services usually are provided either at one or more centrally located health facilities or in the private practice offices of the physicians and other health care providers that are part of the plan. All covered care must be received through plan providers or from other health care professionals to whom the plan refers participants, or else the plan will not pay.

Most plans require individuals to select a primary care physician. The primary care physician is responsible for managing a person's medical care, admitting the person to a hospital, and referring him/her to specialists. Individuals are allowed to change their primary care physician as long as they select another physician affiliated with the plan.

Risk- and Cost-Based Plans

There are two types of HMO contracts with Medicare: risk and cost.

Risk plans. Risk plans have lock-in requirements that specify all the forms of care must be received through the plan or through referrals by the plan. In most cases, unless services are received from an authorized provider, neither the plan nor Medicare will pay. The only exception is for emergency services received anywhere in the United States and for services urgently needed when someone is temporarily out of the plan's service area. Another exception offered by a few risk plans is the point-of-service (POS) option. Under the POS option, the plan permits a person to receive certain services outside the plan's provider network and the plan will pay a percentage of the charges. This additional flexibility by the plan often requires the insured to pay at least 20 percent of the bill. The POS option is a feature of many HMOs and is not limited to

Medicare risk plans. Beginning in 1999, risk contract enrollees will be considered to be enrolled in Medicare+Choice plans, which are discussed in the following pages.

Cost plans. Cost plans do not have a lock-in requirement. When enrolled in a cost plan, a person may go either to health care providers affiliated with the plan or go outside the plan. When services are received outside the plan it will not provide coverage, but Medicare benefits will be payable.

Medicare pays its share of approved charges. The individual is responsible for Medicare's deductibles and coinsurance amounts, just as if he/she were receiving care under the fee-for-service system. The cost plan may be a better choice for someone who travels frequently or lives in another state for part of a year, or wants to use a physician who is not affiliated with the plan.

Health Maintenance Organization (HMO) Enrollment Procedures

Most Medicare beneficiaries have the option to receive Medicare benefits through an HMO. The names of the HMO in an area are available from the state insurance department. To be eligible to enroll, a person:

- must have Medicare Part B and continue to pay the Part B premiums;
- must live in the plan's service area;
- cannot be receiving care in a Medicare-certified hospice; and
- cannot have permanent kidney failure at the time of enrollment.

All HMOs that have contracts with Medicare must advertise open enrollment periods of at least 30 days once a year. Plans must enroll beneficiaries in the order of their application. No one may be rejected because of poor health, with the exception of end-stage renal disease.

If an area is served by more than one plan, individuals may want to compare physicians' qualifications, facilities, premiums, copayments, and benefits to determine which plan best meets their needs. Before making a decision, it is prudent to weigh the advantages and disadvantages of plan membership with other coverages that may be available.

If individuals enroll in an HMO and later decide to disenroll and return to fee-for-service Medicare, they need to send a signed notice to the plan or to their local Social Security Administration office or, if appropriate, to the Railroad Retirement Board. They may return to fee-for-service Medicare the first day of the next month after the plan receives their request to disenroll.

Medicare+Choice Enrollment Procedures

Beginning in 1998 and continuing through 2000, Medicare+Choice beneficiaries will have continuous open enrollment and disenrollment, allowing them to switch plans or move into or out of traditional Medicare. Then, during the first six months of 2001, a transition period takes effect. At this time, beneficiaries may change plans once in addition to during the annual coordinated election period. The annual coordinated enrollment period is to take place each November beginning in 1999. Additionally, beginning January 1, 2001, beneficiaries first eligible for Medicare may switch to traditional Medicare at any time during the first 12 months of enrollment. Beginning in 2003, beneficiaries may switch plans during the first three months of a year, plus during the annual coordinated election period.

Medicare+Choice plans must accept eligible individuals without restriction during election periods (also referred to as open enrollment periods). Enrollment cannot be denied by plans or organizations on the basis of health-status–related factors. The enrollment of a beneficiary may not be terminated unless the person has not paid the premium or has engaged in disruptive behavior or unless the plan is terminated for everyone in the area.

At the time of enrollment and then annually thereafter, each plan must:
- provide specific information to enrollees about plan features, including information on quality of care, utilization review, and the specific procedures for grievances and appeals;

- have a quality assurance program and agreements with an HHS-approved independent quality review and improvement organization;
- protect patient confidentiality concerning beneficiary health information;
- have procedures for physician participation; and
- prohibit "gag" clauses that restrict providers from advising patients about their health status or medical treatment even though the plan may not provide a given treatment.

In addition, plans cannot force providers to indemnify the plan against liability for denial of medically necessary care.

Individuals with end-stage renal disease cannot enroll in a Medicare+ Choice plan. However, an individual can remain in one if diagnosed after enrollment.

Underwriting

There are two types of health underwriting that insurance companies use for Medicare supplements: guaranteed issue (i.e., no health questions are required) and selective underwriting (i.e., health questions are required).

Guaranteed Issue

Guaranteed issue, as the names implies, means that everyone is accepted and will be issued a Medicare supplement policy, regardless of his/her health status. While exceptions may exist, most nonselective underwriting must occur during the open enrollment period. Insurers may use a shorter application form (without health questions) during the open enrollment period.

Selective Underwriting

Selective underwriting requires each applicant to answer a series of health-related questions. Insurers decide—based on the medical information on the application and other medical information received from the applicant's physician(s)—whether to issue the coverage. Some companies may reject an applicant with a serious medical history, such as having cancer, diabetes, heart disease, or a combination of illnesses. Other conditions that may result in the rejection of certain applications include the acquired immune deficiency syndrome (AIDS), drug addiction, or a person currently in a hospital or nursing home.

An applicant's health status is not the only factor to consider when underwriting Medicare supplements. Other factors that could cause an insurance company to reject an applicant for Medicare supplement insurance include:

- a person's Medicare eligibility (a Medicare supplement does not provide benefits unless Medicare pays its portion);
- the age of the applicant in most states (the applicant must be at least age 65 to qualify);
- having other Medicare supplement insurance in force (only one supplement may be in force); and
- being a Medicaid recipient.

Pre-Existing Conditions

Another factor insurers consider when marketing Medicare supplement policies is the length of the pre-existing conditions period. Some companies choose the maximum period—six months—to avoid adverse selection (i.e., tendency of poorer-than-average risks to apply for coverage). Others reduce this period to three or even two months. Some insurers issue policies that protect their applicants from the first day of coverage. The length of the pre-existing–condition period could affect the premium (the shorter the period, the higher the premium), which could affect the competitiveness of the product.

■ Rating

Even though all companies marketing Medicare supplements provide identical benefits in their Plans A through J, premiums vary greatly from one company to another and from area to area (e.g., state to state).

Insurance companies use three different methods to calculate their Medicare supplement premiums: attained age, issue age, and no age (community) rating.

Attained-Age Rates

Attained-age premiums are based on the current age of the insured and increase each year as the insured ages.

Attained-age rates may be calculated based on each individual's age, or premiums may be banded together in certain age groupings (e.g., five-year or 10-year bands). If banded, the premium increases when the insured moves to a higher age band.

For a calendar year, the following is an example of attained-age rates:

Age 65 rate = $ 860
Age 66 rate = $ 880
Age 67 rate = $ 920
Age 68 rate = $ 980
Age 69 rate = $1,020

The following is an example of a five-year age-banded attained-age rate:

Age 65 to 69 = $ 975
Age 70 to 74 = $1,155
Age 75 to 79 = $1,280
Age 80 to 84 = $1,395

Another attained-age rate structure is to increase rates by age up to a certain age (e.g., age 80), after which they remain level. Generally, attained-age–rated plans are initially less expensive than other types of Medicare supplement plans. However, because rates increase as the insured becomes older, over time the premiums will exceed the other types of rating methods.

Issue-Age Rates

When a company uses the issue-age rating method, and the Medicare supplement policy is purchased at age 65, the premium will remain the same. This means that premiums will not increase each year as a person gets older.

Issue-age rates, like attained-age rates, may be calculated based on the individual's actual age at the time of application, or in banded groups.

No Age Rating/Community Rating

Some companies market Medicare supplements by charging the same rate to everyone they insure regardless of their age. This method provides the insured with the simplest way to accurately calculate his/her Medicare supplement rates.

Premium Increases

No insurance company offers a Medicare supplement policy that guarantees its premiums. Over time, premiums for all Medicare supplement plans increase, regardless of the rating method used by the insurance company. Premium increases may be due to a number of factors, including:

- increases in medical inflation;
- higher than anticipated overall claims experience;
- increases in utilization of certain benefits covered by the plan; or
- increases in either Part A or B deductibles and other legislated Medicare benefit revisions.

All Medicare supplement policies and premiums must be filed and approved by the various state insurance departments before they may be sold by an insurance company. Companies may not change their Medicare supplement plans or increase premiums unless the increase is approved by the state insurance department and it applies to all persons in the state covered under the same Medicare supplement plan.

Discounts

Since all Medicare supplement plans provide the same benefits, companies compete with each other on the basis of price and customer service. Some companies use discounts as an incentive for people to buy their Medicare supplement plan.

Spousal Discount

When both the husband and the wife purchase a Medicare supplement at the same time, a company may discount the total premium by a certain percentage (e.g., 10 percent).

Nonsmoker Discount

If the insured has not smoked cigarettes or used tobacco products of any kind (cigar, pipe, chewing tobacco, and so forth) during the past 12 months, he/she is offered a discount. Discounts may range from 10 percent to 20 percent.

Modal Discount

When an insured person pays the full annual premium for a Medicare supplement plan all at once, some companies may discount their premiums by up to 10 percent.

Association Discount

Discounts of up to 20 percent less than an individual premium may be offered by an insurer to each member of an association with a large membership.

■ Regulations

The OBRA-90 required all states to revise their regulatory programs for Medicare supplement insurance. Since then, all states have adopted the model regulation to implement the NAIC Medicare Supplement Insurance Minimum Standards Model Act (see Appendix C), which was adopted in 1991.

The purposes of this regulation are:

- to provide reasonable standardization of coverage and simplification of terms and benefits of Medicare supplement policies;
- to facilitate public understanding and comparison of such policies;
- to eliminate provisions in such policies that may be misleading or confusing in connection with the purchase of such policies or with the settlement of claims; and
- to provide for full disclosures in the sale of health insurance coverages to persons eligible for Medicare.

Major amendments to Medicare supplement regulations enacted since 1990 are discussed below.

Standardized Medicare Supplement Plans

To make it easier for Medicare-eligible persons to compare Medicare supplement insurance policies, all states limit the number of different policies that can be sold to no more than the 10 standard plans described earlier in this chapter. The 10 standard plans do not apply to Minnesota, Massachusetts, and Wisconsin because these states had alternative standardization programs in effect before the federal legislation was enacted and they were not required to change their Medicare supplement plans.

States must allow the sale of Plan A, and all Medicare insurers must make Plan A available if they wish to market any Medicare supplement plans in a state. While not required to offer any of the other nine plans, most insurers offer several plans and some offer all 10 plans. Only two states—Delaware and Vermont—do not allow the sale of all 10 plans. Delaware does not allow the sale of Plans C, F, G, and H. Vermont does not allow the sale of Plans F, G, and I.

Open Enrollment

Federal and state laws provide that for a period of six months from the date a Medicare beneficiary is both enrolled in Medicare Part B and age 65 or older, he/she can buy any Medicare supplement plan regardless of any health problems he/she may have. During the open enrollment period, a person may buy any Medicare supplement plan (even Plan J, the most comprehensive plan offered) sold by any insurer doing business in his/her state. The insurer may not deny the policy because of the medical history, health status, or claims experience of the applicant. Neither may the insurer place conditions on when the policy is issued or becomes effective, nor discriminate in the pricing of the policy, because of the applicant's medical history, health status, or claims experience. The insurer may include a pre-existing condition restriction of up to six months in the open enrollment policy.

The Balanced Budget Act extends the guaranteed issuance of specified Medicare supplement policies to certain continuously enrolled individuals, provided they enroll within 63 days of termination of other enrollment. The table on the following page illustrates this process.

Medicare+Choice Licensing

A Medicare+Choice organization must be organized and licensed under state law as a risk-bearing entity eligible to offer health insurance or health benefits coverage in each state in which it offers a Medicare+Choice plan. A provider-sponsored organization (PSO) must be licensed under state law as a risk-bearing entity to offer health benefits unless the PSO applies to HHS for a license because a state has failed to act on a PSO's substantially completed application within 90 days. If a state has denied a PSO application based on discriminatory treatment or solvency requirements that vary from federal standards, the PSO may apply to HHS. HHS has 60 days to act on the application. PSOs with HHS licenses must comply with state consumer protection and quality standards. After October 31, 2002, PSOs cannot bypass state licensure requirements.

Qualifying Event	For These Reasons	Plans Available for Enrollment
Initial Medicare eligibility at age 65.	Individual enrolls in Medicare+Choice and terminates enrollment during the first 12 months.	All policies (A-J).
Individual terminates Medigap coverage to try Medicare+Choice.	Individual enrolls for first time in Medicare+Choice plan or similar demonstration or Medicare SELECT, and such enrollment is terminated during first 12 months.	Same issuer and same policy as before. (If not available, then plans A,B,C, and F or comparable plans in waivered states.)
Employer coverage ceases.	Plan terminates or ceases all supplemental benefits to individual.	A,B,C, and F (or comparable plans in waivered states).
Medicare+Choice plan enrollment discontinued.	Contract with HCFA terminated; person moves out of service area; plan violated or misrepresented contract; or other per Secretary, HHS.	A,B,C, and F (or comparable plans in waivered states).
Medicare risk, cost, Medicare SELECT, or demo coverage is discontinued.	Contract with HCFA terminated; person moves out of service area; plan violated or misrepresented contract; or other per Secretary, HHS—and, in the case of Medicare SELECT, there is no state law provision for continuation or conversion of coverage.	A,B,C, and F (or comparable plans in waivered states).
Medigap coverage ceases.	Issuer bankrupt or other involuntary termination and there is no state law provision for continuation or conversion of coverage; plan violated contract or misrepresented provisions in marketing.	A,B,C, and F (or comparable plans in waivered states).

Loss Ratio Standards and Refunds or Credit of Premium

A Medicare supplement policy may not be marketed unless it is expected to return to policyholders at least 75 percent for group policies and 65 percent for individual policies. When companies fail to meet these minimum loss ratio standards for each plan offered in a state, they must provide their policyholders with a refund or credit.

Permitted Compensation Arrangements

Insurers may provide commissions (or other compensation) to an agent for the sale of a Medicare supplement policy only if the first-year commission is no more than 200 percent of the commission paid for selling or servicing the policy in the second year or period. The commission provided in subsequent (renewal) years must be the same as that provided in the second year and generally must be paid for a period of no fewer than five renewal years, the length of a renewal period varies by state. No insurer may provide commissions greater than renewal commissions for a replacement policy, unless the replaced policy provides substantially greater benefits than the original policy. *Commissions* means all income payable to the agent including, but not limited to, bonuses, gifts, prizes, awards, and finder's fees.

Required Disclosure Statements

All insurers must provide an outline of coverage to all applicants at the time of application, except for direct response policies (policies sold through the mail), in which case the outlines are included with the issued policy. Medicare supplement outlines consist of four parts: a cover page, premium information, disclosure pages, and charts displaying features of each benefit offered by the insurer. The outlines are required to be printed in a certain sized type and to follow the same format as outlined in the model regulation.

Standards for Marketing

Insurers must establish procedures to comply with the NAIC model regulation. These procedures must provide that:

- any comparison of Medicare supplement policies by an agent is fair and accurate;
- excessive insurance is not sold or issued;
- procedures are in place to determine whether or not a replacement clearly and substantially provides greater benefits (for purposes of triggering first-year or renewal compensation);
- the proper notification—"Notice to buyer: This policy may not cover all of your medical expenses"—is displayed on the first page of every policy;
- every effort is made to determine whether an applicant is already insured by other types of health and accident insurance; and

- auditable procedures are in place to verify compliance with these procedures.

Other marketing practices that have been prohibited include high pressure sales tactics and twisting. Twisting is when an agent induces a policyholder to drop an existing policy to take a similar policy with the agent, to earn a new commission.

Prohibition against Pre-Existing Conditions for Replacements

The NAIC model regulation requires insurers to waive any time period applicable to pre-existing conditions, waiting periods, elimination periods, and probationary periods that the insured has already satisfied under the old policy when the insured is paying for similar benefits under a new Medicare supplement policy. For example, if an insured has satisfied four months of his/her pre-existing-conditions period under one policy, an insurer may not impose more than a two-month pre-existing-conditions period under the replacement policy.

There is a maximum six-month pre-existing-conditions period for all Medicare supplement polices. If a Medicare supplement policy has been in force for more than six months and is being replaced by another Medicare supplement policy, the replacement policy may not impose any pre-existing-conditions period on the applicant.

Summary

Medicare supplements fill the benefit gaps in the federal Medicare program. They provide valuable hospital and medical benefits to millions of Medicare beneficiaries. People need Medicare supplements, and insurance companies try to satisfy this need by offering their products through a variety of different distribution channels, including agents, brokers, mass marketing, employers, and associations.

Congress required all Medicare supplements to be standardized in 1991. Now, customers must pick from 10 plans labeled A though J. Managed care plans available under the Medicare SELECT and Medicare risk contracts are increasing in popularity and are expected to continue to do so.

Everyone is entitled to a Medicare supplement during the open enrollment period, which generally occurs within six months from the time someone first enrolls in Medicare Part B. No insurance company may deny any Medicare supplement policy based on the health of the applicant during the open enrollment period.

Perhaps no other health insurance product has been regulated as heavily as the Medicare supplement. Federal and state requirements control the policy language, benefit structure, loss ratio, commissions, disclosures, and marketing practices. Despite all this, many insurance companies continue to offer one or more Medicare supplement plans to the growing number of people turning age 65.

■ Key Terms

Approved charge
Assignment
Association
At-home recovery
Attained-age rating
Balanced Budget Act
   of 1997
Beneficiary
Benefit period
Calendar year
Charge limitation
Coinsurance
Commissions
Community rating
Deductible

Electronic claims
Exceptions and
   limitations
Excess charge
Guaranteed issue
Issue-age rating
Loss ratio
Mass marketing
Medicare
Medicare Part A
Medicare Part B
Medicare Part C
Medicare+Choice
Medicare supplement
Medicare risk

Medicare SELECT
Model regulation
National Association
   of Insurance
   Commissioners
   (NAIC)
Omnibus Budget
   Reconciliation Act
   (OBRA)
Open enrollment
Pre-existing condition
Selective underwriting
Skilled nursing facility
Underwriting

Chapter 3

HOSPITAL INDEMNITY COVERAGE

63 *Introduction*
64 *Customer Needs*
71 *Benefits*
76 *Underwriting*

77 *Rating*
78 *Regulations*
81 *Summary*
81 *Key Terms*

■ Introduction

A hospital indemnity policy (HIP) is a form of supplemental health insurance that helps protect against loss due to hospitalization. It differs greatly from the more familiar major medical and managed care health insurance in both purpose and characteristics.

- A major medical plan is intended to provide primary protection against significant costs of a major illness or injury. It pays a percentage, usually 80 percent of allowable charges, after the deductible is satisfied.

- A hospital indemnity plan pays a fixed dollar amount for each day a person is hospitalized due to accident only, or accident and sickness. The amount of the daily indemnity can range from $25 (or a minimum established by state law or regulation) to several hundred dollars per day. Unlike a major medical plan, which is an expense reimbursement plan, hospital indemnity pays without regard to actual medical expenses and does not decrease even if benefits are paid by other coverage.

Hospital indemnity coverage originally was designed to be sold to supplement a major medical and/or hospital/surgical plan that paid a specific daily room hospital benefit. In many cases, the plan did not cover the full daily cost of the hospital room. For example, a hospital/surgical plan may have a daily room benefit of $75 and the average cost of a hospital room is $100. In such a case, a hospital indemnity policy would be sold with a daily room benefit of $25.

The need for hospital indemnity coverage has changed with (1) the growth of major medical and managed care plans; (2) the standardization of Medicare supplement plans; and (3) increased costs of medical care. Today's purchaser of a hospital indemnity policy generally already has a major medical or managed care plan that provides coverage for much of the cost of a semiprivate room. This chapter discusses the supplemental benefits provided by a hospital indemnity policy, why it is purchased, and how the policy is sold and regulated.

■ Customer Needs

Gaps in Health Insurance Plans

Hospital indemnity coverage can be used to pay the out-of-pocket costs associated with hospitalization that insureds must pay with a major medical plan. These costs include the deductible, coinsurance, internal policy limits, and medical charges deemed higher than usual and customary. Hospital indemnity also can be used to pay the out-of-pocket costs associated with copayments for enrollees in health maintenance organizations (HMOs). In addition, it covers extra costs incurred due to an illness or injury that are not typically covered by medical insurance, such as travel to a physician or short-term work loss.

Deductibles

Most major medical plans have deductible limits, which require the covered individual to have a predetermined amount of expense for covered treatment before the insurance benefit becomes payable. Deductibles vary by company but typically are based on a calendar year. This means that if an insured has a $100 annual deductible, the first $100 of medical expenses is paid by the individual. Subsequent expenses are covered by the major medical plan. At the beginning of the next year, a new deductible applies and again the first $100 of medical expenses is paid by the individual.

HOSPITAL INDEMNITY COVERAGE

In some plans, the deductible is on a per cause basis, which is the flat amount the insured must pay toward the eligible medical expenses resulting from each illness before the insurance company makes any benefit payments. This means that a specific illness or injury is subject to its own deductible. For example, if an individual with a per cause deductible breaks his/her arm and three months later breaks a leg, the medical expenses associated with the broken arm are subject to a deductible of $250, and the medical expenses associated with the broken leg are subject to a deductible of $250.

Coinsurance

A coinsurance amount refers to the percentage of a covered expense to be paid by the insured after the deductible is satisfied. A typical coinsurance percentage is 80/20, meaning that the insurer pays 80 percent and the insured pays 20 percent of covered expenses. In addition, the insured pays 100 percent of noncovered expenses, such as the amount of an expense that exceeds the usual and customary charge for the treatment or service.

Copayments

Most HMOs include a copayment that applies to inpatient hospital room and board. Plans generally pay 100 percent after a per admission copayment, which ranges from $100 to $500. For example, an individual with a $200 copayment pays the first $200 for each hospital stay, and the plan pays 100 percent thereafter.

Generally, managed care plans also require members to share in the cost of providing medical care. When members visit an in-network doctor, managed care plans typically require that they pay a visit charge, for example, $12 per visit, and if drugs are prescribed, a typical out-of-pocket cost up to $10. Managed care plans also may increase the cost share for members getting care outside the network.

Maximum Out-of-Pocket Expenses

Some plans cap the deductibles and coinsurance limits, providing a maximum out-of-pocket expense. Although this limits the amount of money an individual or family must pay in a calendar year for treatment when hospitalization occurs, it still can be expensive. For example, the cap could be set at $1,000 to $3,000 or more per family. In some cases, the maximum out-of-pocket cost must be met for each insured, not the total family. This approach effectively multiplies the out-of-pocket expense by the number of individuals covered under the policy. Under this scenario, a family of three with a $250 deductible may have to spend $750 per year before the copayment requirement is met.

Internal Benefit Limit

Many types of major medical coverage have an internal benefit limit for all services or for a specific treatment such as mental health care. This maximum payment can be on either an annual or a policy lifetime basis.

For example, a basic major medical plan might have a $250 deductible and a $10 copayment with a maximum out-of-pocket expense of $2,500 per year. The same plan also might limit expenses for mental health treatment and hospitalization to a lifetime maximum of $25,000. If an individual requires hospitalization at $500 per day, is hospitalized for 20 days, and sees an attending psychiatrist each day with an additional charge of $100 per visit, the patient would have already used $12,000, or almost half of the total lifetime benefit, during one course of treatment. Prescription drugs, tests, and other inpatient charges could easily add another $5,000 to the hospital stay. An additional 30 days of psychiatric follow-up or group therapy after discharge would quickly absorb the remaining funds available for not only the initial cause but any other treatments relating to mental health problems at any time in the future.

Usual and Customary Charges

Many health plans, including Medicare, base payment on usual and customary charges. Insurers identify categories of service within a geographic area to determine the average charge by provider or hospital for these services. In the case of Medicare, an approved physician or hospital can charge only up to the fees approved by Medicare. However, when the insured is covered by a private insurance plan, physicians and hospitals can bill for more than the usual and customary charge. This means that there can be a gap between what the doctor or hospital charges the patient and what the insurer provides as a benefit.

Related Expenses

There are numerous other expenses incurred by an insured and his/her family that are associated with a hospitalization. These expenses include:

- travel to and from the hospital, parking, and lodging and meals for family members if treatment must be given away from the home;
- child care during times of hospital visits and possibly in the absence of the primary caregiver;
- long-distance phone calls from the patient's room and from hotels while family members call home; and
- comfort items such as television, newspapers, and comfortable clothing for the patient.

Hospitalization also can bring with it a reduction in income. Not all employers have generous short-term disability or sick leave policies that allow for continuation of income when the employee's absence is due to accident or illness. A short-term disability coverage may have an elimination period of 7 to 14 days, and an insured who was hospitalized may be back at work by the time benefits would be payable. Also, with many two-income families, the loss of even the secondary income could have a significant effect on a family's standard of living. Even if the patient qualifies for continuation of income, the spouse's loss of income during visitation is not replaced.

To help fill these gaps, a hospital indemnity policy pays benefits without regard to and regardless of any other insurance. This means that the benefits provided through such plans can help to:

- pay the deductibles on a calendar or per cause basis;
- supplement coinsurance or copayments;
- offset out-of-pocket expenses;
- provide funds toward noncovered charges;

- pay the difference between usual and customary charges and provider charges; and
- provide funds to offset loss of income of the patient or family members due to hospitalization.

Distribution Methods

Hospital indemnity coverage is marketed through agents and brokers and on a mass marketing basis.

Agents and Brokers

Individual agents and brokers offer hospital indemnity coverage as part of their product portfolios, making it available as a supplemental product to people who have either major medical or managed care plans.

Most of the agent-sold business is handled through work site marketing. Work site marketing is becoming a major way of providing employer-sponsored, employee-paid benefits. In employee-paid, or voluntary programs, the employer contracts with an insurance carrier to provide coverage for employees at group rates. Work site marketing typically refers to voluntary coverage offered to the employee at the place of work by licensed enrollers. Premiums are collected through payroll deduction.

Very few hospital indemnity policies are sold by agents one-on-one with individuals in a person's home. This is due to the decline of individual health insurance sales for these policies. Individual sales declined because most major medical plans cover a semiprivate hospital room, which limits the need to specifically supplement the daily room benefit.

Mass Marketing

The principal distribution channel for hospital indemnity sales is mass marketing. In fact, hospital indemnity policies were the key product that led to the growth of mass marketing in the insurance industry in the 1950s and 1960s. In mass marketing, hospital indemnity policies are offered to the market-at-large or on an endorsed basis.

Broad market sales. Many companies that use mass marketing find hospital indemnity policies to be an attractive product for a large number of purchasers. Once a company obtains a policyholder, it can offer additional health insurance products, such as supplemental outpatient care, rehabilitation, and medical supplies and drugs. To reach a broad market, mass marketers may purchase lists that match demographically with people who purchase hospital indemnity policies. Alternative sales methods such as newspaper inserts, television, telemarketing, direct mail, and radio, also can be used.

Policies distributed through mass marketing methods may have special characteristics, including a special introductory premium and a 30-day no-obligation period in which the applicant can examine the coverage.

Endorsed market sales. The endorsed market includes affinity groups such as associations, clubs, credit unions, and financial institutions. Associations and clubs attract new members by providing them with access to primary and supplemental coverages. Many groups develop a special plan for their members by offering a premium that is reduced to reflect economies in the acquisition and administration of these plans.

The association's insurance broker or internal insurance program administrator usually contacts an insurance company for the coverage. The insurer then offers the product to the membership with the association's authorization. Insurers may be able to include the insurance offer with another mailing by the association, thereby keeping distribution costs low.

Agents associated with banks and credit card companies also may offer hospital indemnity policies to their depositors and credit-cardholders, allowing customers to provide for financial and insurance needs conveniently. A billing vehicle such as a bank account allows the insured customer to make premium payments through automatic deductions and minimizes the potential for inadvertent lapse. The use of billing vehicles such as credit cards makes the purchase of a hospital indemnity policy easy, reduces the number of checks, and saves time and postage for the policyholder.

Customer Service

Hospital indemnity policies are relatively simple to service. Most insurance companies generally have an inbound telemarketing unit to handle policyholder changes. Customer service calls from policyholders typically concern premium amounts and payments, confirmation of benefit levels, and confirmation of coverage for family members. Customer service calls can be used as an opportunity to inform the policyholder of the availability of coverage upgrades.

In many cases the mass marketing insurance company provides a toll-free number to the insured at the time the policy is issued. This enables the insured to call the company with any questions about the features and benefits of the hospital indemnity plan. Since there is no agent involved in a mass marketing sale, these personal calls are important to the policyholder and can help increase the insured's satisfaction and consequently the insurer's persistency and profitability.

Agents also provide customer service to their hospital indemnity policyholders who may need help with a change of address, beneficiary, or mode; adding or removing a spouse or dependent from coverage; obtaining claim forms; or reviewing their coverage.

Automated Service

With the spread of voice-activated or voice-response telephone service, customers can make routine inquiries about their coverage without speaking to a representative. Typical questions concern when the next premium is due, claims status, and premium amounts. Some automated systems allow an insured to update his/her address and telephone number. Increasingly, insureds are using the Internet to update personal insurance information, including change of address.

Premium Payment

The frequency of payment depends on the preference of the insured and the premium alternatives offered by the company. Most companies offering hospital indemnity policies have a wide variety of payment modes, including direct billing annually, semi-annually, quarterly, and monthly. Payment can be made by various methods, such as personal check, money order, electronic-fund transfer, or credit card, subject to state limitations on the use of credit cards. Changes in billing method generally can be done on the telephone with a customer service representative.

■ Benefits

In a basic hospital indemnity policy, a daily room benefit is paid directly to the insured (unless the insured designates that it be paid to the health care provider) for the days of hospital confinement due to injury or illness. Occasionally, accident-only hospital indemnity policies are offered. These plans pay benefits for hospitalization as a result of injury only.

Some plans offer one or more of a variety of benefits, either automatically or at an additional cost, including home health care, an accidental death benefit, surgery, and outpatient medical expenses.

Daily Room Benefit

The core benefit of a hospital indemnity policy is the daily room benefit, which may be payable the first day the insured is hospitalized as a result of sickness or injury. The date that benefits begin varies according to the policy. Some plans do not begin payments until the third day if the insured is hospitalized as a result of sickness. Benefits may range from the minimum required by law, currently about $20 a day, to as much as $400 a day. Many plans on the market provide a minimum of $50 a day.

Given consumer awareness of the high cost of hospitalization and the shortened length of average community hospital stays—from 8.2 days in 1970 to 6.7 days in 1994—several insurers have introduced hospital indemnity plans that provide higher benefits for the first day of hospitalization. The base benefit is doubled for the first day in the hospital. Under such a policy, an insured with a $250 daily room benefit would be paid $500 the first day of hospitalization and $250 a day for the remainder of the hospital stay.

Many plans automatically increase hospital benefits if the insured is hospitalized as a result of cancer or heart attack or is in an intensive care unit, since hospital costs for these conditions tend to be higher.

Benefit Period

Hospital indemnity coverage pays benefits for each day the insured is confined in a hospital. The maximum benefit period can range from 365 days up to life. Since hospital indemnity coverage is sold as supplemental to major medical and managed care plans, hospital indemnity insurers benefit from the risk control measures developed by the primary major medical and managed care companies. Hospitals are aware that primary coverage of hospital expenses will be denied if the patient's stay in the hospital is not medically necessary. Therefore, it is in the hospital's and patient's best financial interest to avoid overlong stays. Coupled with the recent trends to provide more care in a hospital outpatient setting, the risk of providing hospital indemnity benefits beyond the average length of stay is minimized. Some insurers set a maximum level for the benefits the policy will pay, such as $10,000 over a lifetime, or limit the number of days that will be paid on a yearly or lifetime basis.

Intensive Care

Most hospital indemnity policies provide additional coverage for hospitalization in an intensive care unit (ICU). Frequently this coverage is included as part of the basic plan or through a rider issued in addition to the original policy contract. Generally riders pay a multiple of the regular benefit for hospitalization while a patient is confined in an intensive care unit, such as an additional 50 percent or up to double the indemnity amount payable for hospital confinement.

Heart Attack

Many hospital indemnity policies also provide additional coverage for care in a cardiac care unit (CCU). This allows the insured to collect a benefit for critical treatment regardless of the type of service provided by a hospital. In some plans, the greater benefits are paid on the basis of a diagnosis rather than the place or type of treatment.

Optional Benefits

Hospital indemnity coverages frequently include optional benefits such as coverage for outpatient procedures, surgical procedures, recovery time, and accidental death.

- Outpatient procedures: Pays on a per treatment basis. Generally pays a benefit of $25 to $75 after satisfying a deductible of $25 to $50.
- Surgical procedures: Pays either a scheduled or flat rate for surgeries done on an inpatient or outpatient basis; may pay additional benefits for anesthesia.
- Recovery time: Pays a flat daily rate following a qualified hospital stay. Benefits generally are payable for a period of time equal to the hospital stay, and range from $50 to $150 per day.
- Accidental death: Generally provides $10,000 to $100,000 if death occurs within 365 days of the covered accident.

Policy Provisions

Pre-Existing Conditions

A pre-existing condition is defined as a medical condition that normally would have required treatment or advice from a physician and that occurred a specified period of time prior to issuance of the policy. Pre-existing conditions are handled differently in hospital indemnity policies, depending on whether the policies are underwritten.

- All pre-existing health conditions are covered on hospital indemnity policies that are underwritten if the conditions are disclosed on the application.

- Pre-existing health conditions are not covered in policies written as guaranteed issue—that is, offered on a one-time basis without requiring the insured to provide evidence of insurability.

Where there is a pre-existing limitation, the length of time the condition will not be covered varies from 6 to 12 months, depending on the company and the state of issue. For example, under a policy with a six-month, pre-existing condition period, if the insured was treated for a condition within the time frame specified before purchasing the plan, coverage for that condition would not begin until the policy had been in force for six months.

Mental and Nervous Disorders

Most hospital indemnity policies have lower benefits for mental and nervous disorders than for other conditions. Generally the daily room benefit is reduced by a percentage, such as 50 percent, and there is a set maximum number of days paid per confinement, such as 31 days.

Some companies pay full benefits for mental and nervous disorders but have a policy maximum, such as $10,000 over a lifetime, or a maximum total number of days that will be paid for confinement, such as 90 days, with 60 days between stays before a new period begins for confinement. For example, if a person is hospitalized for a mental disorder for 45 days and is readmitted 40 days later, it would be considered as one confinement. If the same person is hospitalized for 45 days and readmitted three months later, it would be considered as two confinements and the insured would be eligible for a full benefit of up to 90 days for the second hospitalization.

Maternity Benefits

Hospital indemnity policies handle benefits for pregnancy in several ways:

- Most policies treat a pre-existing pregnancy the same as any other pre-existing condition. Under this scenario, if the insured is pregnant when the plan is purchased, there is no coverage for that pregnancy.

If the insured becomes pregnant after the purchase of the policy, that pregnancy would be covered.
- Maternity coverage is excluded until the plan has been in force for a period of time—for example, 18 months.
- No maternity coverage is provided.

Benefit Reduction at Age 65

Most hospital indemnity policies provide for a reduction of the daily room benefit at age 65. This adjustment was developed to reflect that at age 65 most Americans become eligible for and enroll in Medicare Part A hospital benefits. (For more information, see Chapter 2: Medicare Supplements.)

Generally benefits decrease by 50 percent, so that if the insured has a daily room benefit of $100 a day, it would be reduced to $50. Since hospitalization increases with age, this reduction helps keep premiums at an affordable level. The need for coverage may decrease at age 65 since in most cases the individual also will have a Medicare supplement plan that pays 100 percent of the Medicare deductible for hospital benefits.

Policy Exclusions

As with all other health insurance products, hospital indemnity policies have several exclusions that vary by state, including the following:

- care that occurs while the policy is not in force;
- benefits for sickness or injury paid under workers' compensation or employer liability laws;
- intentionally self-inflicted injuries while sane or insane;
- loss resulting from the use of taking any narcotic, barbiturate, or other drug, unless administered on the advice of a physician;
- sickness or injury that results from an act of declared or undeclared war;
- sickness or injury sustained while in the armed services;
- nonorganic mental illness; and
- dental care.

SUPPLEMENTAL HEALTH INSURANCE

■ Underwriting

Underwriting of hospital indemnity policies varies according to how they are sold:

- Agent-sold plans usually are underwritten.
- Mass marketing plans usually are guaranteed issue with a provision that pre-existing conditions are not covered for a specified period of time.

Hospital indemnity underwriting is much simpler and not quite as extensive as it is for major medical plans. The applicant's health history is reviewed in less detail since benefits for hospital indemnity plans are limited. The underwriter focuses on the applicant's health history and conditions to see if there is above-average risk of illness that could result in hospitalization.

The underwriter reviews the applicant's medical history, especially medical treatments and the reasons for those treatments over the past 7 to 10 years, and looks for conditions such as high blood pressure, lung or kidney disease, heart or artery disorders, hernia, cancer, arthritis, back disorders, diabetes, digestive disorders, liver disorders, blood disorders, alcoholism, illegal drug use, mental or nervous disorders, or sexually transmitted diseases.

The underwriter also looks at the other insurance coverages the applicant may have with the company to protect against adverse selection and to prevent fraud. Due to the potential for adverse selection, many companies limit the number of policies sold to any one insured.

Occupation and hobbies generally are not a factor in evaluating the risk in hospital indemnity policies, as they are in major medical plans.

The underwriter has several options if the applicant does not fit the criteria for a standard risk. These options include:

- charging an additional premium to cover the additional risk;
- excluding the condition or conditions that increase the chance of hospitalization;

- reducing the benefit level; and
- refusing to issue any coverage.

Rating

On the surface, pricing a hospital indemnity policy seems to be a simple matter since the insurance company pays the insured a specified daily room benefit when the insured is hospitalized. The benefit amount remains level despite medical cost trends, and is increased only with the consent of the insured and the underwriter.

The actuary, however, needs to consider variables such as the number of hospital stays and lengths of stay to evaluate the risk and set an appropriate premium. Also, the actuary must evaluate trends, such as the reduction in lengths of stay. The actuary must review data from a large pool of claimants to arrive at valid assumptions for the future experience of the policy.

Expenses

In pricing a hospital indemnity policy, a major consideration is covering expenses. Expenses include the cost of the distribution system (including compensation for agents and the cost of direct response marketing); issue, administration, and compliance expenses for policy and claims processing; cost of funds; and profit levels.

Another pricing factor relates to the minimum loss ratios required by states. The minimum loss ratio must be accommodated when the company sets its expense and premium levels.

Adverse Selection

Since underwriting varies by method of distribution, assumptions used to determine morbidity costs vary by method of distribution. Products that are underwritten initially have a lower morbidity cost than policies that are guaranteed issue.

Adverse selection must always be included in pricing assumptions for guaranteed issue policies. The antiselection factor reflected in morbidity is affected by the amount of daily room benefits offered. Policies with higher amounts of daily room benefits have worse claims experience because of antiselection. For example, if daily room benefits of $40 and $60 are offered, the $60 daily room benefit will have worse claims experience. If an offering included daily room benefits of $40, $60, and $75, the $75 daily room benefit will have the worst experience, and the $60 daily room benefit will have better experience than it would have had in the first example.

Age and Sex Distribution

Age distribution assumptions are critical in pricing a hospital indemnity policy. Most have age-banded rates. This means that everyone within a certain age group pays the same premium. For example, with five-year age bands, everyone from age 30 to 34 pays the same rate. The same is true for ages 35 to 39, 40 to 44, and so on. This approach tends to produce higher profits at the low end of the age band and lower profits at the high end. Age banding can be important for the long-term profitability of the product.

Sex distribution is another factor in pricing. Females and males have different claims cost histories. For example, younger females of childbearing age may be hospitalized for pregnancy and complications of pregnancy, such as high blood pressure or diabetes. Males tend to be hospitalized later in life due to heart disease.

■ Regulations

Federal Regulations

Federal laws that affect comprehensive medical insurance generally may also affect hospital indemnity coverage.

Omnibus Budget Reconciliation Act of 1990 (OBRA)

Federal law prohibits the sale of insurance to a Medicare-eligible individual where such insurance duplicates benefits the individual is entitled to under Medicare. Under the 1996 changes to OBRA, supplemental health insurance products that pay benefits without regard to other coverage are not considered to duplicate Medicare benefits. Persons applying for such coverage, however, must be furnished a disclosure statement as a part of or together with the application for such a policy.

A disclosure statement was designed for each type of product. The disclosure statement for policies that provide benefits upon both expense-incurred and fixed indemnity bases should be used for hospital indemnity coverage. A sample disclosure form can be found as Appendix E.

Health Insurance Portability and Accountability Act of 1996 (HIPAA)

HIPAA is designed to expand access to health insurance coverage and to make such coverage portable. The act generally applies to plans that provide medical care. It does not apply to plans that provide only a list of "excepted benefits." Hospital or other fixed indemnity insurance is an "excepted benefit."

Other Federal Laws

Other federal laws may have an impact on accident coverage or the offering of such coverage in an employee benefits package. The application of these laws to accident and health insurance is discussed more fully in *Fundamentals of Health Insurance: Part B*.

State Regulations

Hospital indemnity policies are subject to the same filing requirements that apply to other accident and sickness policies. Almost all states require submission of individual policies for review by the department of insurance prior to use. Some states deem a form approved after a specified period, unless the form is disapproved by the state prior to issuance or delivery of the form in that state. Other states require that forms be formally approved by the state prior to issuance or delivery of the form in that state.

When a hospital indemnity policy is submitted for review, the regulator may apply all pertinent laws and regulations applicable to accident and sickness policies in general to that policy.

Minimum Standards

Nearly half the states have adopted a version of the National Association of Insurance Commissioners Individual Accident and Sickness Insurance Minimum Standards Act (Appendix A), which includes hospital indemnity policies. As a result, hospital indemnity policies are subject to the basic standards plus several items that apply specifically to it, including:

- a requirement that the plan provide a daily benefit of not less than $20 per day and a benefit of not less than 31 days per confinement per person.
- a definition of *sickness* that limits the length of the probationary period to 30 days from effective date of coverage;
- a limit of 12 months for the length of time a pre-existing condition can be excluded, unless specifically excluded;
- the requirement that the plan use a standard definition of what constitutes a hospital;
- an outline of coverage requirements; and
- disclosure of this information to the consumer.

Rate Review Standards

Hospital indemnity policies are subject to the rate review standards applicable to accident and sickness policies in each state. Almost all states have a statute that provides that accident and sickness policy benefits must be reasonable in relation to premiums charged. In addition, many states have adopted benchmarks to determine whether benefits provided under a policy are reasonable in relation to premiums charged. Generally, the minimum loss ratio for a policy cannot be lower than 50 percent.

■ Summary

Hospital indemnity policies provide supplemental benefits to cover expenses resulting from the treatment of medical or accidental emergencies in a hospital. In the design and marketing of hospital indemnity coverage, it is assumed that the applicant already carries other health insurance protection. The plans provide benefits regardless of whatever other insurance an individual may have and without regard to actual medical expense or cost share. The benefits may be used for any need the insured or his/her family may have, including deductibles, copayments, expenses not covered by the insured's major medical plan, and loss of income due to hospitalization.

■ Key Terms

Age-banded rates
Adverse selection
Coinsurance
Copayment
Daily room hospital benefit
Deductible
Endorsed markets
Guaranteed issue
Hospital indemnity policy

Internal benefit limit
Major medical
Mass marketing
Maximum out-of-pocket expense
NAIC Individual Accident and Sickness Insurance Minimum Standards Act

Outpatient medical expenses
Payroll deductions
Pre-existing conditions
Pricing
Surgery benefits
Underwriting
Usual and customary charges

Chapter 4

SPECIFIED DISEASE INSURANCE

83 Introduction
84 Customer Needs
89 Benefits
93 Underwriting

93 Rating
94 Regulations
99 Summary
99 Key Terms

■ Introduction

Specified disease insurance is coverage designed to provide extra protection upon the occurrence of a particular type or types of illness or disease. These policies originally were sold to cover losses from polio. With the development of a polio vaccine and the decline in the incidence of the disease, companies began issuing cancer-only policies and specified disease insurance to cover other illnesses.[14]

Specialty risk products for specified diseases are designed to supplement coverage under a comprehensive medical insurance policy and to address nonmedical expenses associated with serious illness or disease. Generally, the coverage provides a cash benefit to the insured that he/she can use to pay medical and related expenses. This type of insurance continues to be popular, and in 1994 the market for specified disease insurance exceeded $1.1 billion in annual premium.[15]

This chapter explains the needs that lead to the demand for this type of product, how policies are designed to meet these needs, and what the related regulatory issues are. Much of the discussion centers on cancer insurance since it is the most prevalent specified disease insurance available in the marketplace today. Other specified disease products cover heart surgery, heart attack, stroke, kidney failure, major organ replacement, brain tumor, multiple sclerosis, paralysis, dismemberment, severe burns, or blindness. Unlike cancer, these conditions generally are provided for in a critical illness policy that pays a lump-sum benefit for diagnosis of any of the conditions.

■ Customer Needs

Serious illness or disease can occur at any time. Cancer, heart disease, acquired immune deficiency syndrome (AIDS), and countless other conditions afflict numerous individuals every day. For example, cancer strikes three out of four American families, and approximately 85 million Americans now living will eventually develop cancer.[16] Even people covered by comprehensive medical insurance may face tremendous financial disruption.

Gaps in Comprehensive Medical Insurance Plans

Comprehensive medical insurance policies generally cover the following costs:

- hospital charges;
- drugs and other medical devices;
- nursing care; and
- surgeon, physician, and radiologist fees.

Such policies may, however, have significant gaps that can leave individuals and families in difficult financial positions when an insured family member is diagnosed with a devastating illness or disease. These gaps are created by deductibles, coinsurance, internal benefit limits, overall maximums, exclusions, and limitations.

Deductibles

Comprehensive medical insurance policies require the insured to incur a certain amount of covered expenses before the benefits become payable. This deductible can be applied on an all-cause basis in which the deductible amount is met by the accumulation of all eligible expenses for any variety of covered claims, or on a per-cause basis in which the deductible is a flat amount the insured pays toward the eligible medical expenses resulting from each illness before the insurance company will make any benefit payments. In either case, benefits derived from a specified disease policy can be used to pay this expense.

Coinsurance and Copayments

Comprehensive medical insurance and managed care plans use a coinsurance arrangement in which the insured is responsible for some portion of the payment after the deductible is met. Managed care plans generally require a copayment when services are rendered by a participating provider as well. A reimbursement percentage is expressed as a percentage of the expenses covered by the insurer (e.g., 80 percent). An 80 percent reimbursement percentage means that the insured is responsible for a coinsurance of 20 percent of the cost. Most policies have an annual limit of out-of-pocket expenses that the insured must pay. Even with that limitation, coinsurance can represent a significant expense for the insured when a serious illness such as cancer is involved.

Internal Benefit Limits or Overall Maximums

Comprehensive medical insurance policies generally have a maximum overall benefit limit. This can be a lifetime limit for all causes or per cause. Serious illnesses such as cancer may exhaust benefits under comprehensive medical insurance coverage.

Exclusions and Limitations

Comprehensive plans also contain exclusions or limitations on medical services and supplies. Expenses associated with such exclusions or limitations often are met by specified disease insurance. Common exclusions or limitations in comprehensive medical insurance plans include:

- blood/plasma/platelets;
- expenses associated with donors (e.g., bone marrow);
- experimental treatments;
- home health care;

SUPPLEMENTAL HEALTH INSURANCE

- hospice care;
- occupational sickness;
- private nursing;
- prostheses; and
- reconstructive and cosmetic surgery.

Related Expenses

Among the significant expenses associated with serious illness or disease are those that are not directly related to the provision of medical care. Often these expenses are not considered when an individual or family assesses the exposure of financial risk that may result from serious illness or disease. These related expenses include but are not limited to travel, lodging, meals and special diets, child care, loss of income, and other personal expenses. Many of these expenses are unavoidable given the prevalence of dual income and single-parent families in our society.

Travel. Serious illness or disease frequently calls for treatment in a city where the patient does not live. Transportation to the treatment location can be expensive, depending on the distance from the patient's home. It is often necessary for a family member to travel to the treatment location as well. Transportation expenses also can arise in situations where a donor (such as a bone marrow donor) is involved in treatment.

Lodging. When outpatient treatment for serious illness or disease is performed in a location other than where the patient lives, both the patient and the family member can incur lodging expenses. Lodging expenses also can arise when a donor is involved in treatment.

Meals and special diets. Individuals whose treatment involves travel also incur restaurant charges and other meal expenses. Additionally, special diets, which can be more costly than normal diets, frequently are an important part of treatment for certain diseases.

Child care. Sometimes the patient is the primary caregiver for a child. In other situations, the primary caregiver may need to travel with a family member who is the patient. With the primary caregiver absent in either case, additional child care expenses often are incurred.

Loss of income. Individuals can best protect their income through disability income insurance. Such policies, however, may have elimination periods of 30 days to 6 months and often replace a maximum of 66 percent of income. Coverage under a specified disease policy would be beneficial in the common occurrence of an employed spouse or parent being required to miss work due to care-giving responsibilities. In that case, the employee would not be disabled and therefore not covered by disability insurance.

Other personal expenses. There are numerous other personal expenses (phone calls, pet care, yard care, and so forth), perhaps unique to an individual, that can contribute to the financial hardship caused by a serious illness or disease.

Distribution Channels

Specified disease insurance is offered through numerous distribution channels and generally is marketed on an individual basis. In fact, individual policy sales account for about 98 percent of the market. As the popularity of specified disease and other voluntary supplemental products increases, the availability of group products may expand. Specified disease insurance is sold through a variety of distribution channels, such as the workplace, trade or professional associations, agents and brokers, and mass marketing.

Workplace

One of the primary methods of distributing specified disease insurance is at the workplace as a payroll-deducted, voluntary benefit. Voluntary benefits are those benefits that an employer offers but the employee selects and pays for. As a voluntary offering by the employer, individual specified disease insurance has proved to be an important employee benefit option. This is particularly true in an environment where employer-provided medical insurance coverage is limited.

Associations

Specified disease insurance is marketed through trade and professional associations and other third-party sponsors such as credit unions. Many people like purchasing insurance products through organizations to which they belong. Some associations or third-party sponsors provide services, such as collecting the premium.

Direct Solicitation

Agent solicitation. Another method of distributing specified disease insurance is direct person-to-person selling through an agent. Policies offered this way can include more complex product designs with a higher level of benefits than policies offered through the mail. An agent can also service a market that cannot be accessed easily through the work site as well as people who prefer using their own agent rather than the insurance company selected by their employer. Sales by agents represent a significant portion of premium for individual specified disease insurance.

Mass marketing. Some carriers use mass marketing to sell specified disease insurance. This method of solicitation reaches large numbers of prospective insureds through the mail or other forms of printed media such as newspapers or magazines. The carrier distributes material outlining the coverage along with a simplified application form. Materials used in this method must be simple and precise, and the application form must be easily completed by the applicant. Plan designs generally are limited and may be subject to more restrictions, such as a greater use of pre-existing–condition exclusions, than plans sold by agents.

Customer Service

As is the case with all insurance products, customer service is an essential element of the value of the product. The ability to deliver policyholder benefits both promptly and accurately is critical. Nationwide toll-free customer service is common among carriers providing specified

SPECIFIED DISEASE INSURANCE

disease insurance. Carriers using mass marketing rely almost totally on their toll-free numbers to provide policyholder services.

Agents and brokers also provide customer services. For example, an agent presentation may include detailed product information or a review of other coverage of the individual seeking specified disease insurance. Carriers that sell through the work site also provide other personalized customer services, such as giving employees information about their employer's overall benefits package. In all instances, a high level of customer service is critical to retaining customers.

■ Benefits

Benefits under a specified disease policy generally are paid:

- without regard to other coverage that the insured has; and
- directly to the insured.

These two features provide the insured with financial resources at the time when the need is critical. Benefit payments must be triggered by some event related to serious illness or injury—either by the provision of some medical service, device, or drug or by the diagnosis of the disease. Some policies may use a combination of these triggers. Many policies provide specialized benefits such as for wellness or screening and for death resulting from the covered illness or disease. Consumers have a wide choice of benefit levels ranging from very inclusive coverage with no lifetime limits to fairly limited coverage. The higher the benefit levels, the higher the premium.

Wellness Benefits

Many specified disease policies contain an annual wellness benefit that is designed to encourage prevention or early detection of the serious illness covered by the insurance. Generally this type of benefit pays a flat fee after the insured has a covered test. Policies frequently provide an additional wellness benefit for a follow-up screening test that resulted from an abnormal result on a previous test.

89

Wellness-related tests that may be covered under a cancer policy include:

- bone marrow testing;
- breast ultrasound;
- CA 15-3 (blood test for breast cancer);
- CA 125 (blood test for ovarian cancer);
- CEA (blood test for colon cancer);
- chest X-ray;
- colonoscopy;
- flexible sigmoidoscopy;
- Hemoccult stool analysis;
- mammography;
- Pap smear;
- PSA (blood test for prostate cancer);
- serum protein electrophoresis (blood test for myeloma); and
- thermography.

Medical Event Benefits

Specified disease benefits often are triggered by medical events common to the treatment of the covered illness or disease. Medical events covered under most policies include inpatient benefits, surgical procedures, nonsurgical treatments, and extended care.

Inpatient Benefits

A daily benefit for confinement in a hospital or intensive care unit for the covered disease or illness is a basic feature of specified disease policies. Other benefits related to a hospital stay that may be provided are for ambulance or air ambulance services, attending physician fees, private nursing services, and drugs and medications that are prescribed while the insured is in the hospital.

Surgical Procedures

Specified disease policies provide benefits for surgery performed for the treatment of the covered disease or illness and for anesthesia used in that surgery. The policies also may include benefits for second surgical opinions, reconstructive surgery, prostheses such as artificial limbs, and wigs for hair loss.

Nonsurgical Treatments

Treatment of certain illnesses or diseases may require nonsurgical treatments. This is clearly the case with cancer. Such treatments include radiation, chemotherapy, antinausea medication, blood/plasma/platelets, and experimental treatments. Experimental treatment can involve hospital, medical, and surgical care.

Extended Care

Often treatment of a specified disease or illness requires follow-up care in a skilled nursing care facility. Other extended care benefits may include family care, hospice care, and home health care services.

Diagnosis Benefits

The diagnosis of the specified disease or illness also is a benefit trigger. Benefits based on diagnosis generally require a pathological diagnosis, but exceptions are made where a pathological diagnosis is not possible, such as in the case of a brain tumor. Diagnosis benefits can be provided in stand-alone coverage or as an additional benefit in a policy that provides medical event benefits.

Lump Sum

Diagnosis benefits generally are paid in a single payment upon the initial diagnosis of the covered disease. The advantage of the lump-sum initial payment is that it gives the insured cash early in the treatment period to help pay for expenses that may arise before other benefits are triggered.

Progressive Payment or Building Benefit

Specified disease policies may contain a provision that increases the initial diagnosis benefit based on the length of time the insured has been covered under the policy.

Death Due to Covered Disease

This benefit is a lump-sum amount paid to the insured's beneficiary in the event the insured dies from the covered illness or disease.

Exceptions and Limitations

A specified disease policy is bound by its nature to provide coverage for named illnesses or diseases. This fact must be prominently displayed on the policy and all related materials; the policy should not be marketed as a substitute for comprehensive health insurance coverage. Within these boundaries, specified disease policies have few exceptions or limitations. Exceptions and limitations that may be encountered include skin cancer and pre-existing conditions.

Skin cancer. Cancer coverage may provide only limited benefits for skin cancer or no benefit at all. Melanoma, although commonly appearing on the skin, may be diagnosed and treated as an internal or more serious type of cancer due to its tendency to metastasize internally.

Waiting periods/pre-existing condition limitations. Specified disease policies may impose either a waiting period or a pre-existing condition limitation period. A waiting period is a specified number of days during which no benefits or a reduced amount are payable under the policy. The waiting period for specified disease policies usually is 30 days. A pre-existing condition limitation restricts coverage for a specified period for conditions present prior to the effective date during a "look-back" period. The length of this limitation varies from state to state and from plan to plan.

SPECIFIED DISEASE INSURANCE

■ Underwriting

Specified disease insurance generally is issued upon completion of a simplified underwriting process. For the most part, risk selection factors are limited to the absence or presence of the covered disease or illness during a defined period up to and including the date of application. For example, the questions about medical history on an application for cancer insurance are generally limited to whether the proposed insured has had cancer, leukemia, Hodgkin's disease, melanoma, or malignant tumors of any kind.

Policies with high benefit levels or policies that cover multiple critical illnesses may require a more extensive underwriting process. In these circumstances, carriers may inquire about additional risk factors, such as family history or health habits. This is particularly true where the likelihood of contracting the covered illness is enhanced by engaging in certain activities (e.g., smoking) or by the presence of another disease (e.g., diabetes and its relation to heart disease). Additionally, many carriers inquire about whether the proposed insured has tested positive for the human immunodeficiency virus (HIV) or has been diagnosed with or received treatment for AIDS.

This simplified underwriting process does not exclude every applicant who indicates a history of a specified disease or illness. In some cases, the insurer may elect to issue the policy with a limitation for a certain condition. For example, an individual may have a history of skin cancer other than melanoma and the carrier may decide to issue a cancer policy with an exclusion for skin cancer. In this event, the applicant would still be able to obtain coverage for internal forms of cancer and to provide coverage for their families.

■ Rating

There are very few differences between the way premium rates are established for specified disease insurance and for other health insurance. Generally, information relative to incidence, costs per incident, persistency, and the expense structure are considered. Age and sex distribution are relevant to claim frequency. Participation levels are important to products sold at the worksite, since higher participation levels lend stability to a block of individual business sold. Other factors that can affect the premium rate include:

- plan design;
- trends in medical care;
- trends in the economy, including inflation;
- extent of underwriting;
- contract renewability provisions;
- regulatory issues; and
- marketing strategies.

Regulations

As with other types of health insurance, there are some federal laws that relate to specified disease insurance, but mostly it is regulated as health insurance under state law. In some instances, however, states have issued regulations that are specific to specified disease insurance.

Federal Regulation

Federal laws that affect comprehensive medical insurance generally may also affect specified disease insurance.

Omnibus Budget Reconciliation Act of 1990 (OBRA)

Federal law prohibits the sale of insurance to a Medicare-eligible individual where such insurance duplicates benefits the individual is entitled to under Medicare. Under the 1996 changes to OBRA, supplemental health insurance products that pay benefits without regard to other coverage are not considered to duplicate Medicare benefits. Persons applying for such coverage, however, must be furnished a disclosure statement as a part of or together with the application for such a policy.

There are two disclosure statements that apply to specified disease coverage. One applies to policies that reimburse expenses incurred for specified diseases or other specified impairments. The other statement is for policies that pay fixed dollar amounts for specified diseases or other specified impairments. A sample disclosure form can be found as Appendix E.

Health Insurance Portability and Accountability Act of 1996 (HIPAA)

HIPAA is designed to expand access to health insurance coverage and to make such coverage portable. The act generally applies to plans that provide medical care. It does not apply to plans that provide only a list of "excepted benefits." Specified disease insurance is an "excepted benefit."

Other Federal Laws

Other federal laws may have an impact on specified disease coverage or the offering of such coverage in an employee benefits package. The application of these laws to health insurance is discussed more fully in *Fundamentals of Health Insurance: Part B*.

State Regulations

The regulation of specified disease insurance varies from state to state just as it does with any other line of insurance. Both group and individual specified disease insurance is subject to the jurisdiction's general regulation of health insurance. These regulations may include the application of standard provisions for health insurance contracts, minimum benefit standards for individual policies, advertising guidelines, and rate regulation, including mandated minimum loss ratios. In some jurisdictions, there may be specific provisions that address specified disease insurance only. The National Association of Insurance Commissioners (NAIC) models discussed below affect specified disease insurance in different ways. Laws and regulations in a particular state may vary from the models.

SUPPLEMENTAL HEALTH INSURANCE

NAIC Minimum Standards Acts and Implementing Regulations

About half of the states have adopted some version of the NAIC minimum standards. These provisions set out minimum benefit requirements, standard policy provisions, and required disclosure provisions for all accident and health insurance. (See Appendices A, B, and C.)

Minimum benefit requirements for specified disease policies depend on the type of coverage in question. The model differentiates between cancer and noncancer coverage and whether the coverage is expense incurred or indemnity. There are specific benefit requirements for:

- expense-incurred cancer-only coverage or expense-incurred cancer coverage in conjunction with one or more specified diseases;
- expense-incurred noncancer coverage;
- per diem indemnity cancer coverage; and
- lump-sum indemnity coverage.

To ensure that the minimum benefit requirements are met, the model specifies that specified disease coverage must be sold or offered for sale as such. Therefore, it is not possible under the model to file a specified disease policy as either a hospital confinement, limited benefit policy, or any other type of supplemental coverage.

In addition to minimum benefit standards, the model imposes certain standard policy provisions. Among the more significant requirements are that the policies be at least guaranteed renewable and that the benefits under the policies be paid regardless of other coverage. There also is a restriction on any waiting or probationary period and on any pre-existing condition limitation. Waiting or probationary periods are limited to no more than 30 days following the effective date. Pre-existing–condition limitations are limited to a six-month look back with a six-month maximum exclusion.

Under the model, specified disease policies are subject to substantial disclosure requirements. In addition to the information that must be included in the outline of coverage, specified disease policies must contain a prominent statement on the first page of the policy in contrasting color or boldfaced type that states, "CAUTION: This is a limited policy. Read it carefully with the outline of coverage and the Buyer's Guide." The Buyer's Guide referred to in the statement must be provided at the time of application. Mass marketing insurers must provide the Buyer's Guide upon request. The outline of coverage must provide similar disclosures. It also must contain a statement that the policy is designed only as a supplement to a comprehensive health insurance policy and should not be purchased unless the person being insured has that underlying coverage.

NAIC Advertising Guidelines

The NAIC Advertising Model Regulations and accompanying guidelines are designed to help carriers accurately represent the benefits provided by specified disease policies and to prevent advertising that tends to exaggerate the risk involved with contracting a particular illness or disease. Key among the advertising requirements is a disclosure statement that clearly and conspicuously states the nature of the policy. For instance, advertisements for a cancer policy must include a statement substantially similar to, "THIS IS A CANCER-ONLY POLICY." Advertisements for specified disease policies also must avoid synonymous terms that imply coverage that is broader than what is actually provided for in the policy. For example, a critical illness policy cannot imply that benefits apply separately for heart disease and for coronary disease. Another example might be the use of the terms HIV and AIDS to imply separate coverage, one for HIV and one for AIDS.

The regulations and guidelines also prohibit the use of terms or phrases that tend to create fear or anxiety. One example provided is, "Cancer kills somebody every two minutes." Such a statement is not permitted if it is made without reference to the total population from which the statistics are drawn. It is permissible, however, to use statistics from an organization such as the American Cancer Society as long as the source is properly documented and the statistics are not overemphasized. Additionally, phrases that overemphasize the risk of financial hardship associated with contracting a disease or illness are restricted; such phrases include *financial disaster* and *financial shock*.

SUPPLEMENTAL HEALTH INSURANCE

The regulation does not allow the use of total benefit maximum limits in a headline or caption unless applicable daily limits and other internal limits are referred to there as well. It also prohibits the mention of total benefit limits when such limits would not be reached on an average claim.

Small Employer Market Reforms

Specified disease products generally have been excluded from the application of small employer and other insurance market reforms. Several states, however, require an annual certification that any specified disease policies marketed in the state are not marketed or sold as substitutes for comprehensive or major medical coverage. California and Vermont require that an application for a specified disease policy inquire about coverage under a comprehensive or major medical policy. If the individual does not have such coverage, the policy cannot be issued. If the carrier complies with the requirements of the small employer law, the question need not be asked. The restriction in these two states only applies to the small employer market.

Sales Restrictions and Limitations

During the late 1960s and early 1970s, there were allegations in several locations concerning improper market conduct practices related to specified disease insurance. These allegations revolved around high pressure sales tactics and related marketing issues. In some instances, the allegations were substantiated and were addressed by the industry. There were, however, some regulatory efforts to address market conduct issues. One example is the Medicare-nonduplication provisions that were included in OBRA. Other efforts resulted in regulatory provisions that either directly or indirectly prevented the sale of such policies. Today, these prohibitions and restrictive provisions are for the most part in the past. Only two states, New Jersey and Massachusetts, continue to have a prohibition or limiting provision.[17]

New Jersey. New Jersey law does not currently allow the sale of specified disease policies, with the possible exception of coverage provided under group policies lawfully issued in another state. The law states that

98

"[n]o policy shall provide coverage for specified disease(s) or for procedures or treatments which are limited to specified diseases."

Massachusetts. Massachusetts also rejects the stand-alone specified disease concept. The Massachusetts regulations require coverage of an extensive list of illnesses or diseases and requires that the coverage only be sold as a supplement to basic hospital insurance. The state also continues to review the status of this product.

■ Summary

Specified disease insurance has evolved over time to address particular diseases or illnesses that have a disproportionately high impact upon individuals and families. Decades ago, polio was such a disease, but with the development of a vaccine, polio is no longer a concern in the United States and most other countries. Today, people are concerned about the serious impact of cancer, heart disease, and AIDS, to name a few diseases. If and when medical solutions are developed for today's concerns, future generations are likely to face the threat of some as-yet-unknown diseases.

Specified disease insurance is well suited to provide protection from the effects of chronic and emerging diseases to individuals who perceive risks beyond those covered by basic insurance. As new viruses and resistant strains of bacteria evolve, so too will specified disease policies to cover those new health concerns.

■ Key Terms

Agent	Copayments	Health Insurance
Association sales	Critical illness policy	Portability and
Benefit limits	Deductibles	Accountability Act
Benefit maximums	Diagnosis benefits	of 1996 (HIPAA)
Cancer policy	Direct solicitation	Inpatient services
Clinical diagnosis	Exceptions and	Loss of income
Coinsurance	limitations	Lump sum payment

SUPPLEMENTAL HEALTH INSURANCE

Mass marketing
Medical event
 benefits
Medical expenses
NAIC Minimum
 Standards Act
Nonsurgical treatment
Omnibus
 Reconciliation
 Act of 1990
 (OBRA)
Pathological diagnosis
Payroll-deducted
 benefits
Pre-existing–
 condition limitation
Progressive payment
Related expenses
Specified diseases
Surgical services
Wellness benefits

CHAPTER 5

ACCIDENT COVERAGE

101 *Introduction*
102 *Customer Needs*
109 *Benefits*
113 *Underwriting*
117 *Rating*
119 *Regulations*
121 *Summary*
121 *Key Terms*

■ Introduction

The original accident insurance policies, issued in the mid-19th century, provided benefits for accidental death or severe injury for railway travelers. Soon after, insurance companies as well as commercial travelers' and railway employees' accident associations and certain beneficiary or fraternal orders began offering accident policies. Today, many companies offer travel accident coverage and travel insurance covering common carriers, motor vehicles, and airplane flights. Over the years, accident insurance has expanded beyond travel to provide protection against loss of life and limb, medical expenses, and loss of wages due to accidental injuries or death that occurs on and off the job.

The difference between an accidental injury and accidental death is always clear. However, it is not as easy to define what an accident is. Most accident policies use the concept of injury. A bodily injury may be defined as an injury to the body resulting directly from an accident and independently of all other causes. This definition normally excludes all diseases, including alcoholism (although it might include alcohol poisoning).

Some insurers have an accidental means clause, which generally covers a loss brought about solely by external, violent, and accidental means. The terms *external* and *violent* indicate an unexpected physical force against the body. Such a clause may require that the claimant show visible evidence of this force. Examples of an incident caused by accidental means are:

- transport or vehicular accidents;
- unintentional poisoning;
- fires;
- lightning, storms, or other natural events;
- being struck by an object; and
- homicide.

The accidental means clause requires that both the cause and the result be unexpected. The terms *external* and *violent* are in addition to the accidental means requirement. Many states now forbid the use of *external* and *violent*. This type of clause has been replaced by "results" language, which refers to the occurrence of an injury resulting directly from an accident and independently of all other causes.

Courts have made a distinction between accidental means and accidental injury. The following are examples of accidental injuries that did not result from accidental means, even though the results may have been unexpected:

- injury while lifting heavy objects;
- injury from medical treatment;
- drug or alcohol overdoses; and
- exposure to medical X-rays.

This chapter discusses the four major types of accident insurance: accident medical expense; accidental death (AD) and accidental death and dismemberment (AD&D); accident disability; and travel accident coverage.

■ Customer Needs

The annual toll of accidents in the United States is staggering. In 1995, the total number of unintentional injury deaths was 93,300, or 35.5 per

Table 5.1

Costs of Unintentional Injuries in the United States, 1995 (in billions of dollars)

Lost wages and productivity	$222.4
Medical expenses	75.1
Insurance, police, and legal administration	73.6
Motor vehicle property damage	36.2
Costs to employers	19.3
Fire losses	8.2

SOURCE: *Accident Facts, 1996.* 1996. Itasca, IL: National Safety Council.

100,000. The total number of injuries that left people disabled beyond the day of injury was 19.3 million. Overall, the annual cost of accidental injuries (including fatal and nonfatal accidents) exceeded $430 billion in 1995. Table 5.1 shows the major components of the costs of accidental injuries.

From an actuarial perspective, most accidental losses are insurable. While accident trend data are not as accurate a measure for predicting losses as are mortality data for life insurance, accident data provide enough accurate information for insurers to determine the probabilities of accidental injury and death by age, sex, and cause.

Accident insurance as a supplement to medical expense insurance is popular for several reasons, including the following:

- Accidents are a leading cause of injury and death for people under age 40. Accident coverage may cover a significant portion of the needs of younger insureds.
- Accidents occur (or at least appear to occur) more randomly than sickness. Even though people can and do mitigate the risk of accidents, it is difficult to completely do away with their occurrence.

Accident Medical Expense

Accident medical expense reimbursement was one of the earliest forms of medical reimbursement. This type of insurance provides for payment of medical expenses following a covered injury. Another type of plan is accident hospital indemnity. It pays benefits based on the number of days hospitalized and is not based on the actual amounts charged. Neither type of coverage is comprehensive. Rather, they are viewed as supplemental coverage for insureds who have major medical policies, partial coverage for those with no health insurance, or additional insurance in the event of an accidental injury.

Deductible and Elimination Period

Accident medical expense policies usually have a zero or small deductible or zero-day elimination period, and begin paying on the first day of hospitalization or treatment due to an accident. Sometimes a policy may cover both accidents and sickness. In such a case, the sickness benefit may have a deductible or elimination period.

Dependents

Accident hospital policies may be written to cover the primary insured, his/her spouse, each child separately, or all children for various benefit amounts. The policy also can be written directly on a dependent child, as in the student/sports accident policies discussed below.

Common Accident Medical and Hospitalization Expense Policies

Common accident policies that provide medical and hospital expenses are accident medical expense policies, accident hospital indemnity policies (AHIPs), and student/sports accident policies.

Accident medical expense policies. There are a variety of plans possible based on the type of events covered. They may cover any accident or they may be related to specific events such as broken bones or outpatient coverage. These policies often are sold by agents as supplements to help pay major medical coverage deductibles.

Accident hospital indemnity policies. Accident hospital indemnity policies are widely sold, particularly in the mass marketing market. They almost always include both a fixed daily hospital benefit and an accidental death benefit. Additional benefits such as ambulance, emergency room, intensive care unit, and scheduled surgery benefits often are provided through riders. These riders may be sold with the original policy or may be added later through rider or upgrade marketing programs.

All-accident or 24-hour accident policies. These are accidental death and dismemberment policies with additional medical coverage tied to actual medical expenses relating to an accident. They usually are sold by agents or through mass marketing methods.

Student/sports accident policies. These policies may provide 24-hour coverage or may cover only school hours plus one hour before and after school. They often provide blanket benefits with moderate limits and specified exclusions, such as organized sports and benefits payable under automobile coverage. Special sports coverages are available to student athletes during organized events. Another variation is camp coverage to provide accident insurance to youths at summer camps. Student and sports accident policies usually are sold on a group basis.

Accidental Death (AD) and Accidental Death and Dismemberment (AD&D)

Accidental death and accidental death and dismemberment provide a lump sum on the occurrence of an accidental death or accidental dismemberment. The amount of coverage is called the principal sum. To determine a connection between an accidental death and an insured accident, there may be a time limit (e.g., 90 days after the accident) by which death must occur to receive benefits. Some AD&D policies provide travel accident coverage as well, in the form of additional benefits for common carrier or automobile accidents.

Accidents on or off the Job

Many AD&D policies cover accidental death or dismemberment regardless of whether it occurs on or off the job.

Accidents While Traveling

Most AD&D policies do not contain a restriction on benefits payable if an accident occurs while traveling in the United States or in a foreign country. However, accidents are difficult to investigate under any circumstances, and the problem of determining payable benefits is even harder in foreign countries.

Accident Disability

Monthly Income When Disabled

An accident disability policy is like any other disability policy, except that benefits are payable only when the cause of the disability is an accident. There are two ways to base determination of disability for accident disability insurance:

- whether the insured could perform the duties of his/her own occupation; or
- whether the insured could perform any gainful activities for which he/she is reasonably suited.

If disability occurs during a period of unemployment, then some established method used by the insurer (e.g., using the occupation on the application for the own occupation definition) is used. Some insurers use a definition of disability based on activities of daily living during a period of unemployment.

Accident disability is sold as either:

- 24-hour coverage, which covers all accidents including those occurring at work and covered by workers' compensation; or
- nonoccupational coverage, which excludes any injuries that are covered by workers' compensation.

The benefit period for disability benefits may be short term (i.e., for a year or less) or long term (i.e., even continuing to age 65). Benefits cease upon recovery, death, or the end of the benefit period. During a

ACCIDENT COVERAGE

period of disability and when an insured is receiving benefits, premium payment often is waived.

Credit Disability Insurance

Credit disability insurance offers coverage for loan payments for insureds who become disabled. Since it covers all causes of disability, not only accidents, it is not covered in this chapter.

Travel Accident

Travel accident insurance covers aviation accidents on scheduled airlines, accidents on other common carriers (including taxis, buses, and subways), and motor vehicle accidents. Scheduled airline coverage is usually on a per trip basis, but other types of common carrier or motor vehicle accident coverage are sold on a monthly or annual basis. Coverage can be for one trip, a short period, or continuous. Travel accident plans may be sold as accidental death coverage with additional medical reimbursement benefits.

Travel accident policies were once very popular for air travel and were sold in most terminals. Although still available that way, they mostly are sold by mass marketing, particularly when the trip and the travel insurance are billed on the same credit card.

Employers offer travel accident insurance as a way to give supplementary accident protection to employees traveling on company business. Some employers provide a comprehensive or all-risk plan, which gives 24-hour protection from the time an employee leaves his/her home or place of business until he/she returns from a business trip. Others limit accident coverage to common carriers, described below. The cost of business trip insurance usually is paid entirely by the employer.

Common Carrier

Common carrier coverage is sold either as a part of travel accident coverages or as separate coverage in an accidental death policy. Common carrier policies cover injury while the insured is a fare-paying passenger

107

on a public carrier operated by a licensed common carrier for regular passenger service. The demand for common carrier coverage is high for several reasons:

- The actual probability of an event occurring is small, and the rates are very low; thus, large amounts can be offered at low rates.
- Many people fear flying.
- Although accidents happen infrequently, when they do occur they may be spectacular and highly publicized.

One Trip/Multiple Trips

Travel accident coverage for air flight covers a one-way trip with no intermediate points, a continuing trip with several intermediate points, or a roundtrip with several intermediate points that returns to the original departure point. A policy for any of these types of coverage is billed on a per trip basis.

Other types of policies with common carrier benefits cover all common carrier accidents and are not billed on an individual trip basis. Instead, they have a fixed monthly premium. The AD&D common carrier benefit covers any number of trips on common carriers in exchange for a fixed monthly premium. In contrast to benefits that charge on a per trip basis, it does not matter how many or how few trips are taken.

Other Travel

Common carriers cover many travel situations, including airlines, cruises, trains, taxis, buses, and subways. Travel accident policies may extend the accident coverage to include:

- any accident on airport premises;
- any accident between two legs of a multiple flight trip; and
- any accident during a short vacation between two legs of a roundtrip flight.

One of the main types of travel accident not covered by common carrier coverage is the private automobile accident. For such coverage, a separate benefit may be issued.

Distribution Channels

Accident insurance is sold either by insurance agents including work-site marketing, or by mass marketing and direct response marketing, including telemarketing.

Agents

Accident policies typically carry a low premium, they are easy to understand, and most agents have accident policies available to sell. Group accident coverage—namely, AD&D coverage purchased by employers for their employees—usually is handled by specialty brokers or consultants.

Mass Marketing

Since accident products typically cost less than $100 per year per policy, they need to be sold in large volume, and both unit expenses and overhead need to be kept low to cover fixed expenses and generate a reasonable profit. Mass marketing can meet these requirements. A good mass marketing program involves having a large database of potential customers with usable demographic information, being able to statistically analyze important profitability factors, and having a specialized marketing production staff and efficient data processing. Telemarketing is a good venue for selling accident insurance. Because it is more interactive, telemarketing usually requires a larger staff than direct mail.

■ Benefits

Accident benefits parallel other health insurance benefits. The difference is that the events insured are related to an accident. Accident medical benefits are like any other supplemental medical benefits, except that they cover only accidental causes. Accident disability is just like other disability except that only disabilities caused by accidents are covered. Finally, accidental death parallels ordinary life insurance except that accidental deaths only are covered.

SUPPLEMENTAL HEALTH INSURANCE

Due to the limited coverage offered, most accident policies are attractive only at a low price. Often, the level of benefits offered is set based on the target premium level.

Accident Medical Expense Policies

Accident medical expense policies pay benefits for medical or hospitalization expense based on the amount of expense billed to the insured. These amounts may be capped by a maximum amount payable per accident. This amount is stated in the policy.

Benefits may include physician and hospital services, nursing care, X-rays, and ambulance services. These benefits may be combined with accidental death, dismemberment, or travel accident coverage.

Accident Hospital Indemnity Policies (AHIPs)

AHIPs pay a stated benefit for each day of confinement due to a covered injury. Maximum benefits may be any amount from $100 per day on upward. Policies may have no elimination period or may have short elimination periods of up to three days. Benefits may be reduced by 50 percent at age 65 or older. These policies are similar to hospital indemnity policies, but pay only for covered accidents. They also typically provide an accidental death benefit (e.g., of $10,000).

Typical riders added to AHIPs are medical expense supplements, common carrier death benefits, scheduled accident supplements, emergency accident supplements, intensive care indemnity, recovery at-home benefits, automobile/pedestrian death benefits, emergency room benefits, and ambulance payment.

Accidental Death/Accidental Death and Dismemberment
Maximum Benefits

Maximum benefits for AD and AD&D range from $1,000 to $100,000 when coverage is for any cause. If benefit amounts vary based on cause,

ACCIDENT COVERAGE

higher benefits may be available for common carrier or automobile accidents. Common carrier benefits are paid while a fare-paying passenger is in a public conveyance operated by a licensed common carrier.

Automobile/pedestrian benefits are paid if the covered person is injured while driving in a private automobile or is struck by or driving for hire a land motor vehicle. A land motor vehicle includes all automobiles—private as well as taxis—and trucks, buses, motorcycles, trains, and subways.

Loss of Life

In case of loss of life due to bodily injury directly and independently of all other causes and occurring within 90 days of the accident, the insured's beneficiary is paid the full principal sum.

Loss of One or More Members

The full principal sum is paid for the loss of two members, or body parts. A member is usually a hand, foot, or eye. Loss of hand or foot refers to complete severance through or above the wrist or ankle joint. Loss of eye refers to the irrecoverable loss of the entire sight of the eye. If only one member is lost, one-half the principal sum may be paid. Sometimes dismemberment is provided alone without an accidental death benefit, and the term *capital sum* is used for the amount payable.

Exclusions

Exclusions, which vary state by state, typically include accidental death or dismemberment due to suicide, intentionally self-inflicted injuries, war, use of narcotics or other drugs, blood alcohol level, assaults or felonies, and disease, bodily or mental infirmity, or any treatment of the above.

Accident Disability
Monthly Income

Accident disability coverage provides short-term benefits up to six months and in some cases a year. To receive the benefits, the insured must show initial and subsequent proof of disability and the need for regular medical care for the disability. Mental and substance abuse-related disabilities may be excluded.

Maximum Benefits

The maximum benefit for accident disability coverage is:

- a set amount, usually $500 or $1,000 per month; or
- related to lost income and cannot exceed a reasonable relationship to income.

Travel Accident Coverage

Travel accident coverage usually offers large benefits for scheduled airline accidents. These amounts can range up to $1 million. The accident must occur during a covered trip. This can be either a one-way trip or a roundtrip. The insured must be a fare-paying passenger and a separate premium must have been paid for the coverage. Children are insured for a lesser amount, around $25,000.

Additional benefits that may be offered are coverage for other common carriers traveling to and from the airport, and accidents occurring at an airport. These may be offered at the full benefit amount. In addition, all other accidents may be covered during the travel period between departure and return for a lesser amount, typically $100,000.

Daily hospitalization benefits may be added for accidental injuries occurring during the travel period.

Exceptions and Limitations

For accident policies, typically no benefit is paid if the injury:

- is intentionally self-inflicted;
- is due to war or act of war;
- is caused by use of drugs unless prescribed by a physician;

- occurs when the person's blood alcohol level is elevated;
- occurs when the person is acting as pilot or crew in an aircraft;
- occurs when the person is in an aircraft not as a fare-paying passenger;
- occurs while committing an assault or felony; or
- is due to disease, infirmity, or medical or surgical treatment.

Some accident policies pay for all of the above except for disease, infirmity, or medical or surgical treatment. This is a way of re-emphasizing that the policy covers accidents and not sickness and disease.

Disability, hospitalizations, or death due to accidents occurring prior to the effective date of coverage are not covered. Some policies may exclude work-related injuries if the insurer wants to coordinate the policy with workers' compensation.

Disability and hospitalization plans may have an elimination period whereby no benefits are payable until the period has passed. The period begins at the date of injury. Hospitalization plans usually have either no elimination period or a three-day elimination period. Disability elimination periods vary widely. An accident plan usually has at least a 14-day elimination period. These regulations help reduce the number of small claims and keep the premium low.

Underwriting

Historically, underwriting of accident insurance was more prevalent than it is now. Today, very little underwriting is required for accident insurance. Certain risks are handled through exclusion. For example, the major risk factor relating to accidental injury is age, and most accident policies have issue-age limits and some have the benefit expire at age 65 or 70. Other risks are controlled by developing a large block of business or by purchasing stop-loss or catastrophe insurance. If a large enough pool of insureds is obtained, factors such as risky hobbies, sports, alcohol use, driving habits, and age become less important. In these situations, the number of exclusions in the policy often are reduced. The trend for accident rates in the recent past has been

SUPPLEMENTAL HEALTH INSURANCE

decreasing, as opposed to most other health insurance where claim costs have been increasing.

Health information is less relevant for underwriting accident coverages than for other health coverages. However, certain medical conditions, such as epilepsy, may cause concern for the underwriter of accident insurance. If medical underwriting is used, accident coverage may be issued at standard rates, with medical risks underwritten up to about 200 percent of standard rates, or it may be denied. If substance abuse, particularly alcohol abuse, is detected, coverage is usually denied.

For accident disability policies, the issue and underwriting process determines whether the amount of income applied for is reasonable in relation to the person's current income.

If there is no underwriting, the insurance company does not select who will be issued coverage from the pool of applicants.

Most accident policies are written on a guaranteed issue and guaranteed rate basis. Guaranteed issue means the insurance is issued without any underwriting. The only possible reasons for denial might be lack of group membership in the case of group insurance or an individual's having exceeded the number of policies or maximum amount of insurance allowed one individual. Often the term *enrollment* is used for guaranteed issue group insurance rather than *application* since no underwriting is done and the person is simply enrolling in the group insurance plan.

Guaranteed rate means the insurance is issued at a guaranteed standard rate. There is no substandard rating. Everyone of the same age and sex would pay the same premium.

Individual accident policies also are issued guaranteed renewable and noncancellable at fixed rates. Guaranteed renewable means that the coverage may not be terminated (canceled) by an insurer and rates are adjustable only by class. Noncancellable means that the coverage may not be terminated by the insurer and the rates cannot be increased.

ACCIDENT COVERAGE

Short-form Application

With little or no underwriting for accident insurance, most insurers use a short-form application. The form for accident insurance indicates the name, address, sex, date of birth of persons to be insured (usually the applicant, spouse, and any children), and beneficiaries. The application might ask a question such as, "To the best of your knowledge and belief are you and each family member to be insured healthy and free of impairment?"

This is usually the minimum information requested to consider the policy underwritten. There may be a question as to whether the new policy is intended to replace any other insurance presently in force. The applicant's occupation may be asked if an occupational exclusion is to be applied in the underwriting process.

Maximum Benefit Limits (Company)

The primary risk when issuing accident coverage is a natural or man-made disaster or catastrophe that could involve many insureds simultaneously. Such situations generally are handled with catastrophe reinsurance, with excess amount reinsurance, or by limiting the amounts of coverages. Maximum amounts for accident coverage may go as high as several hundred thousand dollars per insured, with higher limits (around $1 million per insured) for common carrier coverage.

The maximum benefit amounts need to be considered in the context of company surplus, earnings, and expected claim variance. Since accident coverage is a low-frequency, high-benefit coverage, it has a larger variance in claim amounts than other health benefits. Companies need to compare this variance with the amount of surplus they have available to absorb these fluctuations. Companies also have to compare this variance with the amount of expected earnings to determine the likelihood of claims exceeding revenues. The higher the maximum benefit, the higher the potential variance in results.

115

SUPPLEMENTAL HEALTH INSURANCE

Maximum Benefits Limits (All Companies)

Accident insurers pay without regard to other coverages. They set maximum benefits based on their own companies' requirements. If there is concern about whether a potential insured has too much disability income or hospital indemnity coverage, it could be handled through determination of insurance in force at issue if underwriting is used.

Occupations

Some accident policies—for example accident disability insurance—are occupationally underwritten, with certain high-risk occupational classifications excluded from coverage. Examples of persons who might be excluded are lumber workers, demolition experts, underground miners, and professional athletes. Other classes can be divided by risk level and charged premiums appropriate to the risk.

Sports/Sporting Events

Issue of accident policies may be restricted if the potential insured participates in dangerous sports or avocations. As mentioned above, professional athletes may be excluded from coverage based on occupation. Most of the traditional underwriting procedures regarding avocations are related to controlling the accident risk. Many different types of risks fall under the general heading of avocations. New types of risky activities are always developing. In life insurance, these accident risks usually are handled with flat, permanent extra premiums or denial. They are rarely underwritten in accident insurance.

Other Underwriting Factors

Other factors that might be related to increased accident risk and considered in underwriting accident coverage, usually through an exclusion, are:

- poor driving record, including speeding tickets, prior accidents, driving while under the influence of alcohol, reckless driving, driving with a suspended license, or multiple minor moving violations;
- use of alcohol and/or other substances; and
- aviation risks unless the insured is a fare-paying passenger.

Rating

Rating of accident coverage can depend on several factors:

- whether there are scheduled premium rate increases in the future (e.g., attained-age);
- whether unscheduled rate increases are allowed if the loss ratio deteriorates (e.g., guaranteed renewable);
- whether individual characteristics such as occupation, driving record, and avocations are used in ratings (e.g., underwritten with extra premium); and
- whether any characteristics of the insured are used at all (e.g., community rating).

Accident coverage ranges from highly specific rates (based on the person's age, sex, and possibly other factors with scheduled or unscheduled increasing rates), to one rate for everyone. Questions of equity and antiselection need to be addressed before an insurer determines what type of structure will be used.

Issue-Age Rating

If an accident policy premium is determined when the policy is issued and never changes due to advancing age, then the policy is considered to be rated on an issue-age basis. An advantage of issue-age rating is that the premium is set and there is no need to worry about rate changes.

SUPPLEMENTAL HEALTH INSURANCE

Most accident insurance is sold on an issue-age, guaranteed rate, noncancellable basis. This type of premium structure tends to develop larger reserves, just as whole life develops larger reserves than term life.

Attained-Age Rating

If the accident policy premium increases as the person ages and depends only on his/her current age, the policy is considered to be rated by attained age. This is analogous to pure term insurance. The company has less lapse rate risk since the policyholders are paying their current claim rates each year. Attained-age rating also allows a lower initial rate since there is no need to provide for future higher claim rates. Even if the rates are attained-age, they still can be provided on a noncancellable basis if the increasing rates are set at issue and guaranteed for as long as the policy remains in force.

Community Rating

Sometimes accident coverage is sold on a basis where all persons in the community pay the same rate, regardless of issue age, attained age, sex, or other factors. This is called community rating. It is important to make sure that the variation in claim rates does not vary significantly across the various factors. For example, an insurer would want to make sure that claims do not vary significantly by age if age is not used. This may be the case if the issue ages are limited (e.g., to ages 20 to 60) or if coverages terminate or reduce by half at age 65.

If claim rates do vary significantly by any of the selection factors that are being ignored, then some antiselection should be expected and rates should be closer to those of the higher risk groups.

Lump Sum

Travel coverage usually is billed on a per trip, per person basis. This makes more sense than rating based on individual characteristics since the risks, particularly on airplane travel, are related more to the trip than the passenger.

Regulations

Federal Regulations

Accident insurance is generally regulated by the states, however, the following federal laws should be considered relative to this coverage.

Omnibus Budget Reconciliation Act of 1990 (OBRA)

Federal law prohibits the sale of insurance to a Medicare-eligible individual where such insurance duplicates benefits the individual is entitled to under Medicare. Under the 1996 changes to OBRA, supplemental health insurance products that pay benefits without regard to other coverage are not considered to duplicate Medicare benefits. Persons applying for such coverage, however, must be furnished a disclosure statement as a part of or together with the application for such a policy.

A disclosure statement was designed for each type of product. The disclosure statement for policies that provide benefits upon expense-incurred and fixed indemnity bases should be used for hospital indemnity coverage. A sample disclosure form can be found as Appendix E.

Health Insurance Portability and Accountability Act of 1996 (HIPAA)

HIPAA is designed to expand access to health insurance coverage and to make such coverage portable. The act generally applies to plans that provide medical care. It does not apply to plans that provide only a list of "excepted benefits." Hospital and other fixed indemnity insurance is an "excepted benefit."

Other Federal Laws

Other federal laws may have an impact on accident coverage or the offering of such coverage in an employee benefits package. The application of these laws to accident and health insurance is discussed more fully in *Fundamentals of Health Insurance: Part B.*

State Regulations

The states provide the regulatory requirements. The major areas of state regulation are policy forms, rates, and advertising.

Policy Forms

In most states, accident policy forms, including applications, riders, and endorsements, must be filed with the department of insurance to make sure the forms meet certain requirements, including that they:

- have a renewability provision;
- identify all separate premium charges; and
- are written in an easy-to-understand style.

Some states require accident-only policies to contain a statement that alerts consumers to the fact that this kind of policy does not pay benefits for loss from sickness. This statement must be placed prominently on the first page of the policy in contrasting color or boldface type at least as large as the policy captions.

Advertisements

States may regulate how insurance companies can advertise their accident policies. Advertisements include:

- printed and published material, audiovisual material, and other literature used in mass marketing, newspapers, magazines, radio, TV, and billboards;
- any literature or sales aid used by an insurer, agent, or broker for presentation to the public, including circulars, leaflets, booklets, depictions, illustrations, and form letters; and
- prepared sales talks, presentations, and material for use by agents, brokers, and solicitors.

Advertisements for accident policies are required to be complete, clear, and not misleading or deceptive. They should use clear wording and not insurance terminology. Deceptive words or phrases should be avoided.

ACCIDENT COVERAGE

Words such as *all, complete, full,* and so on should not be used to exaggerate benefits beyond the policy terms. Limitations and restrictions should not be worded in a positive manner to imply that they are benefits. Advertisements for limited policies, such as accident policies, must contain a statement noting that it is an accident-only policy. Finally, mass marketing insurance advertising is not permitted to indicate that the insurance being offered is low cost because no agent will call or because no commissions will be paid.

Other state restrictions on advertising involve testimonials, use of statistics, policy comparisons, identification of the insurer, group policies, introductory offers, and statements about an insurer. Some states require approval of advertising prior to its use.

Summary

Accidental death and injury are insurable events and can be predicted actuarially with trend data just as are other mortality and morbidity rates. Accidents often are thought of as uncontrollable, and this is one of the key elements of the appeal of accident insurance products. In reality, accidents are not completely uncontrollable events. For example, the use of seat belts and air bags has helped reduce automobile-related accidental death rates.

While accident policies have a high acceptance by consumers, it is important that people understand the limits of the coverage they are buying. There are many types of accident policies sold today, and new types of policies and benefits are being developed to fill market needs. Examples of newer types of accident coverage being offered include benefits for paralysis, and home recovery.

Key Terms

Accident disability
Accident hospital
  indemnity policy
  (AHIP)

Accident medical
  expense policy
Accidental death
  (AD)

Accidental death and
  dismemberment
  (AD&D)
Accidental means

SUPPLEMENTAL HEALTH INSURANCE

- Accidental result
- Agents
- All-accident policy
- Attained-age rated
- Bodily injury
- Capital sum
- Common carrier coverage
- Community rated
- Enrollment form
- Issue-age rated
- Loss of life
- Loss of limb
- Lump sum
- Mass marketing
- Maximum benefits
- Minimum required loss ratio
- Monthly income
- Nonoccupational coverage
- One trip/multiple trips
- Principal sum
- Rate filings
- Renewability options
- Short-form application
- Student/sports accident policies
- Telemarketing
- Travel accident
- 24-hour accident policy
- Unintentional injury
- Workers' compensation

CHAPTER 6

DENTAL PLANS

123 *Introduction*
124 *Customer Needs*
127 *Benefits*
138 *Underwriting*

140 *Rating*
143 *Regulations*
144 *Summary*
144 *Key Terms*

■ Introduction

Nine out of 10 Americans are affected by tooth decay, gum disease, and other oral diseases, according to dental industry statistics. Each year 21 million work days are lost due to oral diseases, and 9,000 people die from oral cancer.

In spite of the widespread incidence of dental disease, dental care represents only about 5 percent of total health care costs in the United States. According to the U.S. Chamber of Commerce, American businesses spend between $1,000 and $5,500 per employee on medical benefits, but only $90 to $500 per employee on dental benefits.

Tooth decay, gum disease, and other oral diseases can often be prevented through sound oral hygiene. Dental insurance provides both the impetus to convince people to visit their dentist and the means to pay for it. Over the past few decades, a new outlook has grown regarding the use of group dental insurance. Employers now realize that significant cost savings can be attained when employees are encouraged to use their dental insurance benefits. In addition, employers receive tax advantages for providing dental insurance to their employees. Dental coverage generally is available through group insurance policies. Prepayment plans—dental health maintenance organizations (HMOs)—have grown in recent years.

SUPPLEMENTAL HEALTH INSURANCE

The private dental insurance market has grown significantly, from 6 million Americans in 1970 to more than 124 million today.[18] With this coverage, insureds can visit a dentist at least once a year. This is clearly one of the main reasons why Americans' oral health has never been better. This chapter discusses the full range of benefits provided by dental insurance.

■ Customer Needs

More than 40 million people lack medical expense insurance, but 140 million—more than three times as many—lack dental insurance, according to the National Association of Dental Plans.[19] Only about half of all U.S. employers offer some form of dental coverage to their employees. And of those covered by medical expense insurance—both group and individual—only 35 percent have dental coverage. Currently, individual dental insurance is offered by only a few carriers.

The two main factors in determining whether a person visits a dentist regularly are having dental insurance coverage and personal income. The higher the income level, the greater the chances the individual visits his/her dentist regularly, whether or not there is dental insurance. Insureds are twice as likely to see a dentist than those without coverage. More than 70 percent of those with dental coverage see their dentist at least once a year compared with 51 percent for those without dental coverage.[20]

There is a direct correlation between a higher rate of occurrence of tooth decay and oral disease and the lack of dental insurance coverage. Studies show that the three groups representing the largest segment of Americans without dental insurance coverage—the elderly, the poor, and minorities—have the highest rate of occurrence of untreated and decaying teeth.

The primary focus of dental benefits is on preventive care, which involves regular visits to the dentist. People who see their dentists regularly need fewer treatments for complicated dental procedures. According to the American Dental Association, from 1979 to 1990, periodic dental check-ups increased 12 percent, while extractions and fillings decreased 41 percent and 52 percent, respectively.

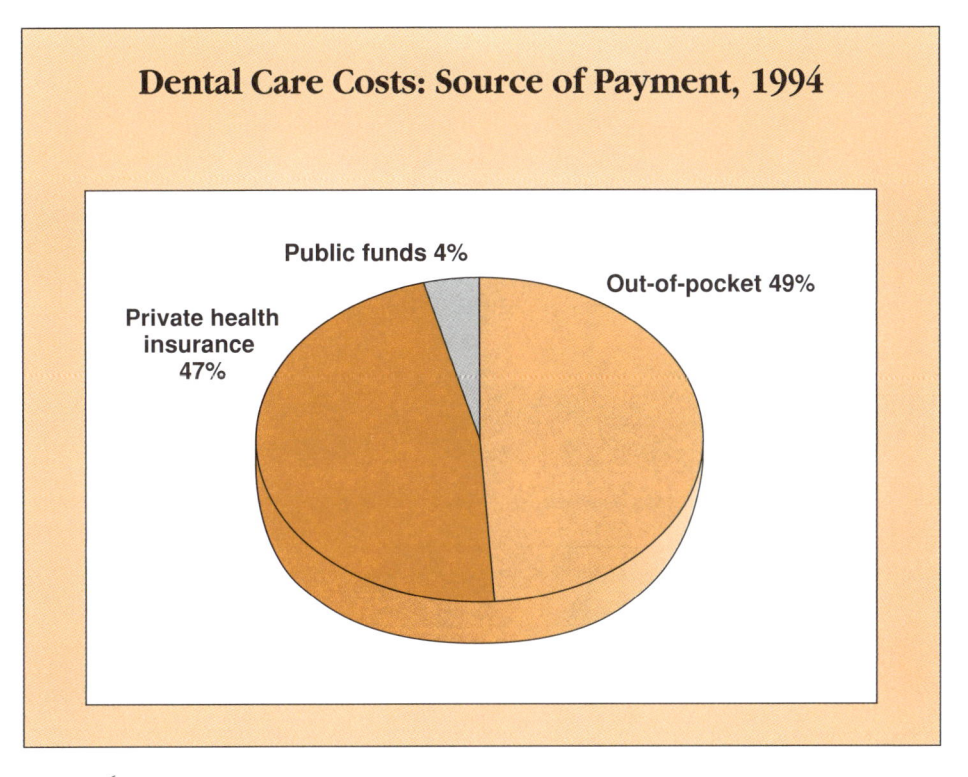

Dental Care Costs: Source of Payment, 1994

- Public funds 4%
- Private health insurance 47%
- Out-of-pocket 49%

Figure 6.1
SOURCE: Health Care Financing Administration. 1996. Health Care Financing Review (spring).

Out-of-Pocket Spending

Because so many people lack dental insurance, out-of-pocket spending for dental care is high. Consumers spend approximately $40 billion annually on dental care, and out-of-pocket payments account for 50 percent of that amount.[21]

Gaps in Traditional Group Coverage

Figuring out the perfect formula for offering good comprehensive employee benefits to attract and maintain a quality work force has perplexed employers for years. Employers have found that dental benefits

SUPPLEMENTAL HEALTH INSURANCE

Dental Plans by Employer Size

Employers with dental plans

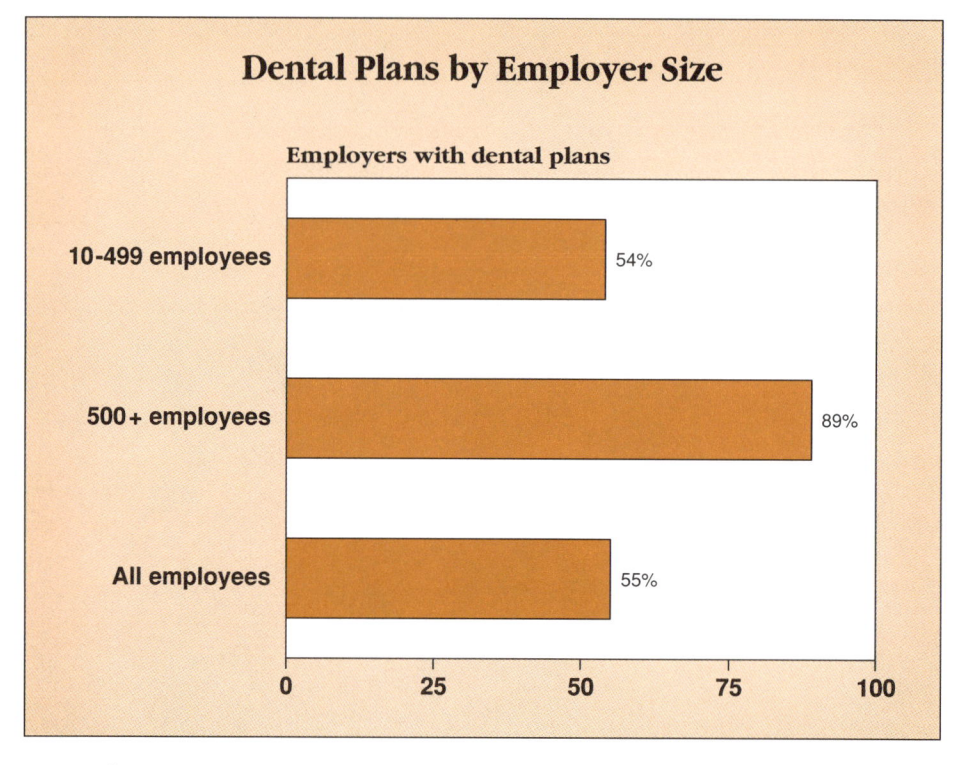

- 10-499 employees: 54%
- 500+ employees: 89%
- All employees: 55%

Figure 6.2

SOURCE: Foster Higgins. 1996. National Survey of Employer-Sponsored Health Plans.

are easy to understand and are appreciated by their employees. In recent years, dental insurance has been one of the fastest growing employee benefits. It is one of the few benefits that can be regularly used without being sick or injured.

Most large employers have added dental coverage to their employee benefit package, but fewer small- and medium-sized employers offer this benefit.[22]

Covered Charges

Dental benefits are designed to share responsibility with the insured for the normal cost of care. The amount of cost assistance provided by the plan varies from plan to plan depending on the purpose and the budget of the sponsor.

Dental insurance contracts specifically detail what is and is not covered. Covered procedures generally include any treatment, service, or materials prescribed by a dentist that are:

- necessary and appropriate;
- nonexperimental or noninvestigational; and
- not in conflict with accepted dental standards.

Treatments or services that are primarily cosmetic generally are not covered expenses. Other charges that generally are not covered are discussed later in the chapter.

Benefits

Dental Plans

As with medical expense insurance, dental insurance is offered in several ways. The prominent dental insurance plans available on the market today are:

- fee-for-service indemnity plan: A traditional plan in which insureds freely choose providers and are reimbursed following the submission of claims for each dental service.
- preferred provider organization (PPO): An arrangement in which a third-party payer contracts with a network of dentists to furnish services at lower-than-usual fees in return for prompt payment and a certain volume of patients. Insureds still have the option to choose a dentist not in the network. However, they may have to pay any dental charges over what would have been reimbursed if they had chosen a dentist in the network.
- exclusive provider organization (EPO): A form of managed care in which participants are reimbursed for care received only from affiliated providers. A dental EPO requires insureds to visit a network dentist or receive no benefits.

- dental HMO: A prepaid health plan that provides dental care services to enrollees within a geographic area, accepts responsibility for delivering services for a fixed periodic rate based on the number of insureds, and is organized under state law as a dental HMO.
- referral discount plan: Insureds are provided a list of providers who charge reduced fees.
- voluntary plan: An employer-sponsored, employee-paid insurance. Insureds get the pricing of a group policy, while the employer pays no part of the premiums. The premium is paid through payroll deduction.

Integrated and Nonintegrated Plans

The dental plan is either integrated with other medical expense coverages or written separately from other coverages (nonintegrated).

Integrated plans. Dental expenses under an integrated plan are blended into the covered expenses of a major medical benefits plan. Generally, coverage is on a reasonable and customary or nonscheduled basis. The deductible must be satisfied each calendar year by either or both medical and dental care expenses. The amount payable for dental and medical care expenses usually is subject to the same coinsurance percentage. Sometimes dental care expenses are separated into classes or categories of services (restorative, prosthodontics, orthodontics, and so forth), and a different coinsurance level is applied to each class.

Nonintegrated plans. Dental expenses under a nonintegrated plan are covered separately from medical expenses as a stand-alone coverage. Dental plans covering the vast majority of employees are on either a scheduled or nonscheduled basis.

Scheduled. Scheduled plans list specific dental procedures similar to a surgical schedule for medical plans. Reimbursement toward the dentist's charges is up to the amount specified in the schedule for each procedure. For example, the insurance plan might pay $40 for a cleaning and $75 for a scaling and root planing. The insured would be responsible for paying any balance over the amount listed in the schedule.

Table 6.1

Sample Dental Benefits

Covered charges	Deductible*	Coinsurance	Maximum benefit**

Preventive procedures including
  Routine exams
  Teeth cleaning
  Fluoride treatments (under age 16)
  X-rays
  Sealants (under age 16)
	$0	100%	$1,000 per person per calendar year

Basic procedures including
  Restorations
  Root canal therapy
  Fillings
  Periodontal scaling
  Biopsy of oral tissue
	$25	80%	$1,000 per person per calendar year

Major procedures including
  Crowns
  Fixed bridges
  Inlays and onlays
  Periodontal surgery
  Full or partial dentures
  Bridge and denture repairs
	$25	50%	$1,000 per person per calendar year

Orthodontic procedures including
  Formal, full-banded retention
  Removable or fixed appliances
  Orthodontia (child only)
	$0	50%	$1,000 lifetime maximum

*Calendar year deductibles for preventive, basic, and major procedures can be combined or kept separate.
**Maximums for preventive, basic, and major procedures are combined.

Nonscheduled. Nonscheduled dental plans are written to cover the percentage of reasonable and customary charges. Nonscheduled plans generally include deductibles, coinsurance, and maximums based on different classes of procedures. Basic services generally are set up to reimburse 100 percent for preventive and diagnostic services, 80 percent for basic procedures, and 50 percent for major procedures such as crowns, bridgework, and orthodontic services. Table 6.1 illustrates the covered charges, deductible, coinsurance, and maximum benefits for a nonscheduled dental plan.

Accident Coverage

Most dental insurance plans cover accidental injury to natural teeth (excluding any injury that occurs from chewing). When the insured's medical expense plan covers accident-related dental services, there is a coordination of benefits and the medical plan generally pays first.

Exceptions and Limitations

Dental insurance generally has frequency limitations for certain services (one oral examination every six months) as well as exclusions (cosmetic-only dentistry). Other limitations or exclusions may include:

- any treatment, service, or material that is not considered as necessary dental care;
- any treatment, service, or material that does not meet professionally recognized standards of quality;
- drugs or medicines, other than antibiotic injections;
- instructions for plaque control, oral hygiene, or diet;
- bite registration or occlusal analysis;
- treatment or service for the purpose of duplicating a prosthetic device or replacing any such device that is lost or stolen; and
- treatment or service that is temporary.

Dental Services

Dental insurance plans are categorized into four general groupings for purposes of plan design. The first three parts are standard; the fourth part is optional.

- Part 1: Preventive/diagnostic services;
- Part 2: Basic services, including simple restorations (fillings), endodontic, periodontic, and oral surgery services;
- Part 3: Major services, including restorative (crowns, inlays, onlays, veneers) and prosthodontic (dentures, bridges) procedures; and
- Part 4: Orthodontics.

Frequency of services provided can vary from plan to plan. Table 6.2 illustrates one company's approach.

Table 6.2

Sample Frequency of Dental Services

Diagnostic
Examinations—one every 6 months

X-rays
Bitewings—one set every 12 consecutive months (6 months if less than age 18)
Periapicals—one set every 6 consecutive months
Full mouth surveys—one in any 60 consecutive months
Panoramic—one set in any 60 consecutive months
Cephalometric—one in any 6 consecutive months

Preventive
Prophylaxis—one in any 6 consecutive months
Fluoride treatments—one in any 12 consecutive months (for dependent children)
Sealants—one in any 36 consecutive months (for dependent children)
Space maintainers—applicable only to dependent children

Restorative
Fillings—replacements covered only if 24 consecutive months have passed since initial filling
Inlays/onlays/crowns/veneers—covered only if the tooth cannot be restored by a filling and (for replacements) at least 84 consecutive months have passed since the last replacement

Prosthodontics
Bridges/dentures—covered only if the teeth being replaced were not missing prior to the effective date of dental insurance; replacements are payable only if the existing bridge is more than 84 consecutive months old.

Oral Surgery—as needed

Periodontics—varies from 3 months to 36 months depending on the procedure

Endodontics—as needed

Orthodontics—generally coverable if bands or appliances were set after the effective date of dental insurance

Diagnostic

In dentistry, diagnostic services are used to determine the existence of dental disease or to evaluate the condition of the mouth. These services include oral examinations, X-rays, clinical and laboratory tests, study models, and photos. They can help in the early diagnosis of tooth decay, gum disease, and oral diseases. Two of the most commonly used diagnostic procedures are examinations and X-rays.

Examinations. Regular exams catch dental problems early, which can lead to less costly dental services. For example, it costs considerably less to fill a small cavity than to build a crown to replace a tooth.

X-rays. There are several types of X-rays used by dentists that are covered under dental plans. The most common are:

- bitewings: intraoral films showing the coronal portions (crowns) of several upper and lower teeth on one film; used primarily to detect decay between the teeth and new decay around old fillings and at bone level; generally taken in sets of two or four;
- periapicals: an intraoral film that shows a whole tooth including root and tissue;
- full mouth surveys: a set of X-rays that shows the entire mouth;
- panoramic: an extraoral film that shows all the teeth on the upper and lower jaws; and
- cephalometric: an extraoral film that shows the skeletal pattern.

Preventive

Thanks to various types of preventive dental care, cavities continue to decline. In 1960, the average American over age 65 had just seven of his/her original teeth. Today, according to Project Hope health researchers, the average 65-year-old has 18 of his/her original teeth. People born after World War II can expect to have at least 24 teeth left when they reach 65.

Sound dental insurance coverage stresses prevention and early treatment. For every dollar invested in dentistry, $8 to $50 are saved. These services are aimed at preserving and maintaining dental health. The basic preventive services include:

- prophylaxis: the professional cleaning of the teeth; smoothes surfaces, removes stains, tartar and deposits, and polishes the teeth;
- fluoride treatments: a procedure to prevent tooth decay; hardens tooth enamel through topical application of fluoride;
- sealants: a procedure to prevent tooth decay; application of resin or plastic to cavity-prone areas (grooves, pits, and fissures) of bicuspids and molars; and
- space maintainers: devices to keep adjacent teeth in place when a deciduous (baby) tooth is prematurely lost so that the space is held

open until the permanent tooth is ready to erupt; either fixed or removable, unilateral or bilateral, depending on the location of the missing teeth.

Restorative

Restorative or operative dentistry is the repair or restoration of teeth due to caries (cavities), trauma, impaired function, abrasion, or erosion. The teeth are restored to regain form and function and to improve appearance. Restorative dentistry can be in the form of fillings, inlays, onlays, crowns, and veneers.

Fillings. Fillings can be accomplished with one of many materials. The two most common are amalgam and composite.

Amalgam. The metallic content of amalgam makes the restoration very strong and allows the restored tooth to stand up to the pressures of chewing and grinding. Amalgam is an alloy made of silver, mercury, tin, copper, and zinc and is the most common form of all fillings. Amalgam fillings have a dark metallic color that contrasts with the color of the teeth and generally are placed in posterior teeth due to their appearance.

Composite. Composite is a plastic material that matches natural tooth color well. It is used most often in anterior teeth for appearance reasons. Composite is not as strong as amalgam, and generally is not a good choice for posterior teeth.

Amalgam and composite fillings usually are anchored to the tooth by a procedure called pin retention. This tiny threaded pin is driven, screwed, or cemented into the prepared cavity and the filling is placed around it. The pin provides additional strength and stability to a large filling.

Inlays. Inlays are used primarily to restore the same type of cavities as silver amalgam. An inlay fits inside or between cusps and is cemented into place. It is essentially a gold filling.

Onlays. Onlays are used to restore teeth with extensive structural loss and undermining of cusps. The interior portion is similar to an inlay, but the onlay casting also has a metal layer that covers the cusps. This is called capping or shoeing the cusps. This serves to strengthen the entire tooth as does a crown.

Crowns. Crowns are used primarily for heavily filled, badly broken, or severely decayed teeth. In such cases, the remaining tooth structure is weakened and the usual filling material cannot withstand forces or add strength to the tooth. Coverage with a crown provides a strong casting that holds a weak tooth together. Crowns also are done for cosmetics reasons, restoration of bite, and occlusion.

The crown is placed over the tooth to hold it together. There are several types of crowns on the market today. The most common are:

- gold;
- porcelain;
- nonprecious metal;
- semiprecious metal;
- resin; and
- porcelain fused to various metals.

Veneers. A relatively new procedure to veneer or laminate the tooth involves etching the tooth enamel with an acid to provide an adhesion of the composite filling material (usually porcelain) to the tooth surface. This procedure is used to strengthen a weakened tooth more conservatively than through the placement of a crown.

Prosthodontics

Prosthodontics is the art of replacing missing natural teeth and tissues with a device or appliance. Although modern dentistry's major objective is to save teeth, extractions sometimes are necessary. Also, teeth may be missing as a result of an accident, congenital defects, or surgery.

Teeth are replaced in a variety of ways. A dental prosthesis is said to be complete (full) if it replaces all of the teeth of a dental arch. A prosthesis is partial if some natural teeth in the arch remain. Prosthetic appliances are either removable, if the patient is to take them in and out; fixed, if they are cemented to the remaining teeth; or implants.

The principal advantage of a partial over a full prosthesis, and the reason it may be worth heroic efforts to save a few teeth, is that a partial prosthesis is attached to natural teeth. If well made, it has the stability and retention that a full prosthesis does not have. This is especially true for the lower arch.

Most carriers do not cover tooth implants, which can cost more than $1,000 a tooth.

Oral Surgery

Oral surgery is the branch of dentistry that deals with the diagnosis and surgical management of oral diseases, injuries, and defects of the jaw and associated structures. Technically, any cutting procedure in the oral cavity is oral surgery and may be performed by any licensed dentist.

Removal of teeth is the most commonly performed oral surgery procedure and is in the top 10 most commonly reported of all dental procedures. Routine extractions are often performed by general dentists as well as by oral and maxillofacial surgeons.

The procedure of tooth extraction ranges from simple to complex. Extractions are divided into three groups: ordinary extractions, surgical removals, and removal of impacted teeth.

Ordinary extractions. Ordinary extractions are referred to as uncomplicated, or simple, and are accomplished by grasping the tooth with forceps and applying controlled pressures that result in removal. Besides forceps, an instrument called an elevator is also used as an aid in tooth removal. Most extractions are of the uncomplicated type, and sutures usually are not required.

Surgical removal. A surgical extraction is necessary when it is not possible to elevate or grasp the tooth to remove it. In some cases, the clinical crown has been completely destroyed by decay or injury, or the roots are crooked or divergent. A tooth also may be fused to bone instead of the periodontal ligament. These difficult extractions are often anticipated, especially in elder patients.

Removal of impacted teeth. The term *impacted* indicates a tooth that is trapped below the gum or bone, unable to erupt. The most commonly impacted teeth are the third molars, or wisdom teeth. Partially erupted teeth are prime areas for infection and can lead to severe pain and swelling. Unerupted or totally impacted third molars may cause pressure, pain, crowding of other teeth, development of tumors or cysts, and damage to adjacent teeth or the jawbone.

Periodontics

Periodontics is a dental specialty that deals with the prevention, diagnosis, and treatment of diseases of the structures that surround and support the teeth. Periodontal disease, commonly referred to as gum disease, is progressive but preventable. It affects 9 out of 10 adults during their lifetimes. Contrary to what most people believe, gum disease, not tooth decay, is the major cause of tooth loss in adults.

Periodontal disease often goes untreated as it can be symptomless, especially in the early stages. Some of the symptoms that can occur include:

- pain and pressure;
- red and swollen gums;
- bleeding;
- bad taste and breath;
- loose teeth;
- sensitivity to heat and cold; and
- movement of teeth from their normal position.

Periodontal procedures include both nonsurgical and surgical procedures. The objectives of periodontal treatment are to teach and motivate the patient to use preventive oral hygiene (brushing and flossing) to restore the health of the surrounding and supporting structures of the teeth.

Endodontics

Endodontics is the specialty that deals with the diagnosis and treatment of diseases of the tooth pulp and associated periapical areas (around the end of the root). Years ago, it was fairly common for a badly broken down and/or painful tooth to be extracted. Today, endodontic therapy is a highly successful and widely accepted method of saving such teeth.

The most well-known procedure in this category is root canal therapy, used to remove the source of infection and to allow drainage. This procedure removes all of the pulp tissue, which is made up of blood vessels and nerves that occupy the pulp chamber and root canal inside a tooth. Once properly prepared and disinfected, the canals are filled with an inert material such as a tin cementing paste.

Orthodontics

Orthodontics is the area of dentistry that deals with the study and supervision of the growth and development of teeth and their arrangement in the mouth. It is the oldest recognized dental specialty. It includes the preventive and corrective treatment for irregularities in the alignment of teeth. The objective is to give the patient a proper occlusion (bite) and "pleasing" facial contour. This is achieved by the repositioning of the teeth by functional or mechanical means.

Any irregularity in the way teeth fit together is called a malocclusion. If left uncorrected, it adversely affects dental and general health, as well as personal appearance. If the teeth are out of position, they are more difficult to clean. This increases the potential of tooth decay and gum disease. Other adverse results include abnormal wear of teeth, speech problems, and emotional problems due to an unattractive smile.

Orthodontic treatment may be preventive, interceptive, or comprehensive.

Preventive. Preventive orthodontics include the use of techniques and appliances that protect what appears to be normal occlusion. Space maintainers are an example. Other preventive orthodontic procedures include early diagnosis of tooth decay and extraction of primary teeth that are late in shedding. Preventive action may reduce the need, or better prepare, for future treatment.

Interceptive. Interceptive orthodontics are procedures that serve to head off or lessen the severity of a developing problem. In addition to the preventive techniques, an interceptive program includes the timely extraction of certain teeth (usually primary teeth), minor tooth movement appliances, or other appliances.

Comprehensive. Comprehensive orthodontics employs procedures to reduce or eliminate an existing malocclusion. These procedures are broad in scope, technically complex, and are most likely to require that the dentist have special training.

Removable appliances are generally made of acrylic and metal or all metal. They resemble a temporary partial denture without teeth. They often incorporate clasps, wires, springs, or expansion screws to provide retention, guidance, support, and desired pressures. These are used more often for preventive and interceptive situations but may be used for comprehensive treatment as well. Retainers and some space maintainers are also considered removable orthodontic appliances.

Fixed appliances, also known as braces or bands, are most commonly used for comprehensive cases. However, there are times when they are appropriate for preventive and interceptive treatment as well.

■ Underwriting

Whether written alone or integrated with a medical plan, dental coverage requires special underwriting considerations for several reasons.

- ■ Dental treatment offers alternative ways of handling a specific condition that can vary in cost (e.g., fixed vs. removable bridgework or gold vs. nongold inlays). An underwriter can give multiple quotes, depending on the plan provisions.

- The range of charges by dentists has a much larger spread than charges for medical care and treatment by medical doctors.
- Many dental charges and even the procedures themselves can be deferred, giving the insured person the opportunity to select against the plan's provisions.
- Many dental expenses, such as capping or some orthodontic treatment, are partially or wholly cosmetic, and thus are elective in nature.

Special Limitations on New Plans

Because dental insurance is not as widespread as medical care expense insurance, a particular group may not have prior experience on which to base rates. When an employer introduces a new dental program, employees who have been lax in proper dental hygiene often have accumulated, and seek correction of, major problems.

This pattern of behavior can lead to extraordinarily high use of the plan in its early years, and it is a major concern to an underwriter. The situation may be even worse when a policyholder announces a new dental plan many months before the effective date and employees postpone all but emergency care until then.

To help offset these factors, the underwriter might request that special limitations be put into a new program, such as:

- a reduced annual maximum to limit the insurer's liability and simultaneously encourage less costly treatment;
- a lower coinsurance percentage for those types of expenses that are either optional (such as gold material) or that are not a part of normal annual maintenance costs;
- incentive coinsurance, which provides a lower coinsurance factor (such as 60 percent in the first year), with subsequent increasing percentages in each year to encourage insureds to spread out claims;

- an advanced approval requirement, often called a pretreatment plan, whereby the employee is required to submit the proposed treatment and its cost for prior approval by the insurance carrier if anticipated costs exceed a certain amount, such as $200;
- the inclusion of a provision basing the benefit on the least costly alternative treatment as determined by the insurer, based on a review of the pretreatment plan;
- a longer eligibility period before the employee can be insured for dental benefits or receive coverage for expensive procedures; or
- a limited benefit for late entrants.

Pre-Existing Conditions Limitations

Another major underwriting consideration is the treatment of pre-existing conditions. A major concern is the expense associated with the replacement of teeth extracted prior to the effective date of dental coverage. These conditions can be handled in a variety of ways. The most common are:

- excluding pre-existing conditions;
- treating them as any other condition;
- subjecting them to a time period (for example, no benefits are covered for 24 months); or
- covering them on a limited basis or subjecting them to a lifetime maximum.

Rating

In general, insurers compute dental expense rates in a manner similar to computation of premium rates for other health care expense coverages. Included in these considerations are type of plans, deductibles, coinsurance, maximums, and covered services.

When rating a small group plan, an insurer's basic rate manual is applied to the group's characteristics. For larger groups, insurers typically use an experience rating formula to adjust their manual rates for prior claims experience. On very large accounts, insurers may give full credibility to actual claims experience. The rate-determination process involves the underwriter evaluating the risk and establishing the proper premium rates.

In establishing the premium for an individual dental plan, the insurer considers plan design as well as marketability. Individual plans tend to have more restrictive limitations than group plans because of the potential for adverse selection. More restrictive benefits can keep the cost of insurance attractive. If the annual premium is greater than an individual's projected annual costs, then that person likely will decline the offering.

There are no exact answers to the problems that arise in establishing premiums. Each underwriter makes decisions based upon his/her years of experience and the company's standard underwriting guidelines.

Factors Considered in Rating

The characteristics of a group or individual are important rating factors that affect the cost of dental insurance. Many insurers look at a variety of considerations when rating a group, including prior dental coverage and specific characteristics of the people to be insured.

Prior Dental Coverage

One factor some insurers take into account when rating a group is whether that group had an existing dental plan. Some insurers have introduced decreasing premium rates for plans that had a previous dental insurance plan. This step is based on the assumption that the existence of a prior plan indicates a lower proportion of needed dental care than is needed for a group that had no prior dental plan, where there is likely to be a pent-up demand for dental services.

If there was no prior dental insurance, some insurers adjust initial rates to cover the expected claims from catch-up dental care. Other insurers may reduce benefit levels for certain major procedures (crowns, bridges, dentures) or exclude those procedures for some period of time. These adjustments to rates or benefits recognize that participants tend to postpone needed dental treatment when there is no insurance coverage.

Finally, because dental treatment often is elective and the potential for selection against the plan is greater than for most coverages, some insurers apply a loading on plans that are written on a contributory basis.

Demographic Factors

Other factors that affect dental rates include, but are not limited to, the following:

Age. The older people get the higher the incidence of high-cost dental procedures. For this reason, age-rating factors generally are used.

Gender. Gender affects dental rates. Females have higher utilization and average claim costs than males. For example, one study showed that females averaged 1.9 visits to the dentist per year, compared with 1.7 for males. Most experts believe that there is not a larger need for dental care among women, but that women are more aware of the need for good dental hygiene than men.

Location. Dentists' normal fees and practice patterns vary from one geographic area to another. For example, the cost of a filling could be substantially different between Ames, Iowa, and Los Angeles. Similarly, certain procedures may be used more in one area than another. The presence of fluoride in the water supply is also important (recent studies show that tooth decay is greater in areas that do not have optimal fluoride levels). For these reasons, area factor adjustments sometimes are used in rating.

Income. The higher the income level, the greater the chance of better oral hygiene habits and use of higher cost services. Also greater dental care accessibility in higher income neighborhoods can lead to more expensive dentists.

Occupation. Studies show that white collar groups generally use their dental benefits more than do blue collar employees. For this reason, industry factors may be used in rating dental plans.

■ Regulations

Compared to medical expense insurance, there is very little regulation that is specific to dental insurance.

Federal

Currently, there is no federal legislation covering dental insurance as a stand-alone product. It is excluded from federal law as an "excepted benefit." (See the discussion of the Health Insurance Portability and Accountability Act of 1996 [HIPAA] in the *Fundamentals of Health Insurance: Part B* and previous chapters in this book.) The most common areas under discussion at the federal level regarding health care reform are uniform national standards, consumer choice, access, due process for patients and providers, consumer rights to health plan information, and quality improvement. While most of these issues have to do with medical expense insurance, the dental industry is monitoring the situation closely for any possible impact on the delivery and payment of dental care.

State

More than half the states have adopted legislation affecting dentistry. For example, many states have mandated dental benefits as a part of the state-mandated medical plans. In addition, dental plans are incorporated into some states' small group reform legislation—for example, portability, community rating, and medical savings accounts (MSAs).

Portability

This provision allows employees who leave their employer-sponsored dental plan to continue group-rate coverage for themselves, spouses, and others by paying premiums directly to the insurer.

Medical Savings Accounts (MSAs)

Dental plans can be included in a medical savings account, a demonstration program that gives tax advantages under certain circumstances.

SUPPLEMENTAL HEALTH INSURANCE

■ Summary

The dental insurance market has grown substantially over the past 25 years, yet with only about half of the U.S. population covered for dental care, dental insurance has not yet reached its full market potential. As more and more employers try to attract and maintain a quality work force, it is predicted that the dental insurance market will continue to grow. That anticipated growth is in contrast to other insurance products that have saturated markets, with little or no pure growth expected (e.g., more than 90 percent of workers in medium and large firms participate in employment-based life insurance plans).

Voluntary dental insurance plans are an attractive market for small employers, especially those that have not offered health or dental plans. Although only a few carriers offer individual dental plans today, individual coverage may be the answer for the millions of Americans who do not have a group voluntary plan or dental insurance provided by an employer-paid plan. As needs change, the dental insurance industry will continue to develop the most appropriate vehicles to deliver the necessary dental care.

■ Key Terms

Basic services
Dental exclusive provider organizations (EPOs)
Dental health maintenance organizations (HMOs)
Dental insurance
Dental preferred provider organizations (PPOs)

Diagnostic services
Endodontic services
Fee-for-service indemnity plans
Integrated plans
Major services
Nonintegrated plans
Nonscheduled plan
Oral surgery
Orthodontic services
Periodontic services

Pre-existing condition
Pretreatment plan
Preventive services
Prior dental coverage
Prosthodontic services
Referral discount plans
Restorative services
Scheduled plan
Selective/nonselective
Voluntary plans

CHAPTER 7

SPECIALTY PLANS

145 *Introduction*
148 *Customer Needs*
149 *Benefits*
158 *Underwriting and Rating*

159 *Regulations*
161 *Summary*
164 *Key Terms*

■ Introduction

There are numerous specialty plans that provide insureds the opportunity for extra health care coverage, in addition to the supplemental products discussed in previous chapters. Examples of specialty plans are prescription drug plans, vision care plans, and TRICARE supplements. TRICARE replaced the Civilian Health and Medical Program of the Uniformed Services (CHAMPUS) in 1997. This chapter focuses on prescription drug plans, and gives an overview of vision care and TRICARE supplements.

Prescription drug plans started as a relatively limited benefit, and often were included as a part of medical coverage. (See the box on limited benefit plans on the following pages.) They now offer comprehensive benefits with varied plan designs and unique administration. Early prescription drug plans generally required an insured to submit a claim form to be reimbursed for prescription drug expenses. These plans also required payment of substantial deductibles or coinsurance payments before any benefits were payable. The average cost of prescriptions was low then, and there was little management of pharmacy-related benefits. Pharmacy claims generally were reimbursed at the prevailing regional rates.

Limited Benefit Plans

The term limited benefit plans has two meanings among supplemental industry insurance professionals. First, it is often used as a general description of all noncomprehensive health insurance products including those covered in this text. Regulators often use the term limited benefit plans whereas insurers tend to refer to this category as supplemental insurance.

The other common meaning of the term comes from the National Association of Insurance Commissioners (NAIC) Model Regulation to Implement the Individual Accident and Sickness Insurance Minimum Standards Act. (See Appendix B.) In this model regulation, the various mainstream individual products are defined with respective minimum standard rules. These include basic hospital expense, basic medical-surgical expense, hospital confinement indemnity, major medical expense, disability income protection, accident only, specified disease, and specified accident coverage. There is also a more general category titled limited benefit health coverage.

In this context, a limited benefit plan is any policy or form (other than specified disease, which must meet the requirements of that section) that does not meet the minimum standards provided under the model. This gives the regulator the authority to approve plans that either fall below the minimum standards of the listed types of individual insurance plans or some type of individual health insurance product that does not fall into one of these categories. If a plan is approved by the regulator as a limited benefit plan, it must contain certain disclosure requirements (see Appendix E). The term limited benefit plan as used in this discussion relates to the category of coverage, limited benefit health coverage.

Purpose of Limited Benefit Plans

A limited benefit plan protects against loss due to accident or sickness. This category of coverage is important because it gives

(continued)

regulators some flexibility in approving new and innovative accident and health insurance product designs that may not meet the standards established for the conventional categories of coverage. Without this category, regulators could have trouble allowing insurers to respond to consumer needs.

Distribution Methods

Limited benefit plans are marketed through agents and brokers or mass marketing. The policies are available through payroll deduction or on direct billing. Payments can be made by various methods, including check, money order, electronic fund transfer, or credit card.

Types of Policies

There are two primary circumstances where a regulator may need to approve a policy as a limited benefit plan. Specifically, a regulator may determine that a proposed policy best meets consumer needs by varying from the standards for the conventional categories. Additionally, there could be changes in a governmental or other comprehensive plan, creating the need for a totally new product design. Both of these events could be addressed under this category of coverage.

Regulations

Limited benefit policies are subject to the same filing requirements that apply to other accident and sickness supplemental policies. Almost all states require submission for review by the insurance department prior to use.

Limited benefit policies are subject to the rate review standards applicable in each state. Almost all states have a statute that provides that limited benefit policy benefits must be reasonable in relation to the premiums charged. Additionally, many states have adopted benchmarks to determine whether benefits provided under a policy are reasonable in relation to premiums charged.

SUPPLEMENTAL HEALTH INSURANCE

In the late 1950s and early 1960s, employers began developing pharmacy networks and prescription drug cards; by the early 1970s, many insurers were managing the networks as a means of reducing claim processing expenses. The growth of drug card programs led to the development of pharmacy claims processors who specialized in pharmacy network management. Manual pharmacy claim forms were replaced by computerized claims processing at the point of sale.

As prescription drug costs rose, employers, managed care organizations, and insurers demanded more complex and varied benefit designs, sophisticated technological support, improved reporting capability, and clinical expertise. This chapter discusses how prescription drug insurance operates in this environment.

■ Customer Needs

Drug costs have been increasing at the rate of 10 percent to 15 percent a year, and this rate of growth is expected to continue. This increase is due in part to the rapid growth in the number of new drugs coming to the market.

Although the growth rate in drug costs is significant, it is important to realize how increases in drug costs affect the total health care budget. For the first time, medical tests have shown that, by increasing the amount of money spent on drug therapy for certain conditions, it is possible to decrease the remaining medical expenses associated with uncontrolled disease. Keeping a patient with medical complications out of the hospital by using a new drug therapy that is more expensive than traditional treatments can have a positive impact on overall health care costs.

Individuals and Families

The primary goal of a prescription drug plan is to meet the needs of individuals and families through optimal health care and the availability of appropriate drug therapy. Health care plans usually offer a variety of prescription drug plan benefit designs to meet the special needs of customers. Plans often include a retail pharmacy program for short-term prescription needs (up to a 30-day supply) and a mail-order pharmacy program for long-term maintenance prescription drugs (up to a 90- or 100-day supply).

Employers

Employers want health care plans that control the costs of providing health care coverage to their employees. Prescription drugs used to represent a relatively small portion of total health care costs. However, prescription drug costs today are a much larger portion of the total health care dollar, and prescription drug plans are receiving a greater amount of attention from employers as a result.

The challenge facing most employers is to balance their desire to control costs with the needs of their employees for prescription drug benefits. While affordability in a plan is important, an inexpensive plan that does not meet employees' needs is ineffective.

Distribution Channels

Prescription drug insurance is marketed to individuals and to employers and organizations that offer group insurance. Plans are marketed to customers by agents and brokers who are contracted to or employed by the health care plan.

■ Benefits

There are two basic types of prescription drug plans: reimbursement and service. Reimbursement plans rely on the insured to pay for any prescription drug ordered and to submit these expenses to the insurer on a claim form. Payment is made to the insured based on the plan agreement. In service plans, payment is made by the insurer to the provider for the product covered by the plan without the insured filing a claim form; the insured usually is required to make a small copayment for each prescription drug ordered. An effective benefit design seeks to provide the optimal drug therapy available while managing prescription drug costs.

Cost Sharing

A prescription drug benefit often requires that insureds share in the cost of the drugs. This cost sharing can include the use of copayments, deductibles, and maximum benefits.

Copayment

A copayment is a portion of a prescription drug expense that insureds pay out-of-pocket to the pharmacy when they purchase a prescription. The copayment usually represents a small percentage of the total cost of the drug. For example, insureds may pay a $15 copayment to the pharmacy at the time they purchase a prescription.

Deductible

A deductible is an amount of prescription drug expense that insureds pay out-of-pocket each year before any prescription drug benefit is payable. When a plan includes a deductible, insureds pay 100 percent of all drug costs until a certain dollar amount is reached. Once the deductible is paid, the benefit plan covers the cost of prescription drugs for the remainder of the year.

Maximum Benefit

The maximum benefit often is referred to as a stop-loss. When a plan includes a maximum benefit, prescription drug costs are covered until a certain dollar amount is reached. Once prescription drug claims exceed this limit, insureds are responsible for 100 percent of the drug costs. Monthly or annual maximum benefit limits may be established.

Covered Prescription Drugs

A prescription drug is any medication or medicinal substance that (1) is approved by the Food and Drug Administration (FDA) and (2) can only be dispensed according to a prescription drug order, under federal or state law. A prescription drug order is a request for a prescription drug by a physician or other health care practitioner licensed by the state to prescribe medications. The pharmacy dispenses a prescription based on the prescription drug order.

Prescription drugs include brand-name and generic drugs; both types are covered by prescription drug plans. In contrast, over-the-counter drugs, which are medications approved by the FDA as safe and effective for self-medication, are available without a prescription and are not covered under prescription drug plans.

Brand-Name Drugs

A brand-name drug is a medication approved by the FDA for the treatment of a certain medical condition. Brand-name drugs have the manufacturer's trade name for the drug on the prescription label.

When a new drug enters the market, it is protected by a patent for several years. This patent guarantees exclusive rights to the drug to the company that produced the medication. When the patent expires, other companies can market the drug under a generic name. A brand-name drug often costs more than a generic drug because other companies cannot market the drug under a generic name until the patent for the brand-name drug expires.

Generic Drugs

A generic drug is a medication that has the same active ingredients as its brand-name counterpart. Generic drugs are approved by the FDA. Many generic drugs can be obtained at a cost savings of 50 percent or more over the brand-name drug. Most companies that make brand-name drugs also make generic drugs.

The use of generic drugs is the single most effective means of controlling drug costs while ensuring appropriate care. Although not all drugs have a generic equivalent, a significant number of generic drugs are available.

Because of the potential cost savings, many prescription drug plans recommend or require generic substitution. Generic substitution is a prescription drug plan provision that requires that a generic drug be substituted for a brand-name drug when an FDA-approved generic drug is available. Some plans may require a higher copayment for a brand-name drug than for a generic drug to encourage the use of generic drugs when they are available.

Dispense as written (DAW). When a physician requests that an insured receive a brand-name product rather than the generic, it is referred to as dispense as written (DAW) enforcement. Depending on the benefit design, insureds may have to pay more for a prescription with the instruction to dispense as written. A plan may require insureds to pay either the difference in cost between the brand-name and generic drugs or the entire cost of the drug when a generic drug is available.

Maximum allowable cost (MAC). Some medications, such as generic drugs, are available from several companies at a range of prices. To standardize the pricing of these drugs and encourage pharmacy networks to make cost-effective drug choices, a health plan may develop a maximum allowable cost (MAC) list. The MAC list, which is distributed to participating pharmacies, gives the maximum dollar amount a pharmacy is paid for a particular generic drug. The MAC price usually is lower than the cost of the equivalent brand-name product.

Exceptions and Limitations

Prescription drug plans may not include benefits for specific services, such as:

- drugs or medicines that can be lawfully obtained without a physician's prescription (over-the-counter drugs);

- drugs limited by federal law to experimental or investigational use;
- drugs for which there are no FDA-approved uses; and
- drugs prescribed for cosmetic purposes.

Formularies

Health care plans often use a drug formulary to ensure appropriate drug therapy. A formulary is a list of the most commonly prescribed medications that have proven to be safe and effective in the treatment of certain medical conditions. Physicians often refer to a drug formulary when writing prescriptions.

Drug formularies have existed for decades. Almost all hospitals have them, and increasingly health care plans are using them. Drug formularies include brand-name and generic drugs. The same drug formulary is used for prescription drugs purchased through mail order as those purchased through local retail pharmacies.

A formulary typically is created by a committee composed of pharmacists, physicians, and nurses who serve as advisors to a health care plan regarding the safe and effective use of prescription medications. The committee decides which drugs are to be included in the formulary, based on current medical literature and the results of controlled clinical tests of the drugs. The committee continually reviews and updates the formulary.

The cost of drugs is a secondary consideration when selecting drugs for a formulary. However, when two drugs are found to be equally effective, the more cost-effective drug may be chosen for the formulary.

The committee may limit the number of drugs within a specific category that appear on the formulary. If a physician writes a prescription for a drug that is not listed on the formulary, the pharmacist can contact the physician to request that a clinically equivalent drug on the formulary be substituted for the nonformulary drug. This is known as therapeutic substitution.

A formulary can be open, incentive, or closed.

- An open formulary is administered on a voluntary basis. Physicians are encouraged to prescribe medications on the formulary, but neither the insured nor the physician is penalized if the formulary is not followed.
- An incentive formulary may provide higher prescription drug benefits for drugs that are listed on the formulary to give insureds an incentive to purchase these drugs rather than nonformulary drugs.
- When a closed formulary is used, an insured who chooses to purchase a drug not on the formulary pays the entire cost of the drug.

Pharmacy Benefit Managers

As prescription drug costs have risen, many pharmacy claims processors have expanded their services to become pharmacy benefit managers (PBMs). Full-service PBMs provide all the services needed to support a prescription drug benefit, including:

- pharmacy network management;
- on-line pharmacy claims processing;
- specialized telephone customer service support;
- mail-order pharmacy services;
- pharmacy benefit design;
- formulary development and management;
- drug utilization evaluation;
- contracting with drug manufacturers;
- drug management reporting; and
- outcomes studies.

The number of PBMs has grown rapidly in recent years as the demand for improved management of drug benefits has increased. PBMs contract with insurance companies, managed care organizations, and employer groups. Some PBMs are owned by pharmaceutical manufacturers.

Pharmacy Network Management

PBMs generally maintain a nationwide network of independently owned and chain-store pharmacies. Many PBMs offer mail-order prescription drug distribution in addition to their retail pharmacies.

Pharmacy standards. To participate in a PBM's national network, a pharmacy must accept discounted reimbursement rates and satisfy the PBM's standards for participation. Each PBM establishes criteria for participation in its pharmacy network. Typically, pharmacy participation criteria include:

- licensing;
- standards for the collection of data;
- compliance with laws and regulations;
- professional, malpractice, and liability insurance coverage requirements;
- acceptance of the PBM's drug management provisions; and
- auditing and quality assessments.

Pharmacy payment. Network pharmacies agree to dispense prescription drugs at rates that are discounted from the average wholesale price (AWP) of a drug. The AWP is the published suggested wholesale price of a drug. A PBM typically pays a network pharmacy the AWP of a drug, less an agreed-upon percentage.

In addition to the discounted payment for the drug cost, the pharmacy receives a professional services fee called a dispensing fee. The dispensing fee is paid to a pharmacy for services it provides, such as patient counseling. A typical formula used to reimburse pharmacies for prescription drugs is:

Example: pharmacy payment = AWP − 10% + $3.00 dispensing fee

On-line Claims Processing

Network pharmacies have on-line, computerized access to information on an insured's eligibility and benefits through the network manager. The pharmacist enters information from the insured's identification card into the computer system along with the drug information from the prescription. The pharmacy computer verifies eligibility, confirms benefits, evaluates potential adverse drug interactions, calculates the appropriate pharmacy reimbursement rate, and determines the insured's copayment.

The pharmacist dispenses the prescription to insureds and collects any copayment from them at the point of sale. The pharmacy is paid for the remaining prescription drug cost by the network manager at an agreed-upon rate.

Mail-Order Pharmacy Services

Many prescription drug plans include a mail-order pharmacy program. Mail-order pharmacy is a method of dispensing medication directly to insureds through the mail by means of a mail-order drug distribution company.

When using a mail-order pharmacy, insureds mail their prescription to the pharmacy, along with any copayment they owe. By using a mail-order program, insureds can purchase a larger supply of prescription drugs, usually up to a 90- or 100-day supply.

Because insureds can receive a larger supply of drugs, a mail-order program often is used to purchase long-term maintenance drugs. A maintenance drug is a prescription drug taken to treat a chronic condition. Examples of maintenance prescription drugs include medications for high blood pressure, diabetes, high cholesterol, heart disease, and arthritis.

A prescription drug plan may include incentives to encourage insureds to use the mail-order program. Subject to state regulations, these incentives could include:

- requiring a smaller copayment amount for a prescription drug ordered through a mail-order pharmacy than for a similar supply of the drug purchased at a local retail pharmacy; or
- allowing insureds to order a higher number of days' supply for a reduced copayment amount, as shown here:

	Supply of drug available	Copayment amount
Local pharmacy	up to 30 days' supply	$15.00
Mail-order pharmacy	up to 90 days' supply	$30.00

Trends in Cost-Effective Plan Management

Pharmacists play an important role in the management of a prescription benefit program. In addition to reviewing drugs for a formulary, they establish criteria for appropriate therapy for different diseases and monitor for appropriate drug utilization. Based on medical literature, they establish guidelines to ensure the safe and effective treatment of several chronic diseases.

Disease State Management

One trend in the management of health care is the concept of disease state management. Traditionally, health care costs have been approached in a fragmented fashion. Pharmacy costs were not associated with overall medical costs for services such as physician office visits and hospitalizations. With disease management, the effectiveness and cost of all of the care used to treat patients with chronic diseases is considered.

As drug costs rise in response to new technologies and the rapid increase in new drugs on the market, these costs must be considered as a part of the total health care dollar. A new drug may manage a chronic disease more efficiently than drugs that have been on the market longer, thereby reducing hospital costs and overall medical costs. By including disease state management programs within a prescription benefit program, a plan can assess total costs and provide positive medical and economic results for its insureds.

Quality Assessment

Health care plans continue to evaluate and design their prescription drug programs to meet increasing consumer demands for quality, and accreditation organizations are incorporating pharmacy services into their performance evaluations.

A key challenge in meeting customers' demands for quality will be to review prescription drug information together with medical information from other sources. In this way, prescription drug therapies can be properly aligned within the overall scope of patient care to ensure effective, quality health care.

Financial Incentives for Physicians and Pharmacies

Responding to the pressures of increasing drug costs, health care plans initially focused on reducing administrative costs, using market leverage to obtain discounts from pharmacy networks, and shifting a portion of the costs to the insured. Although modestly successful, these strategies were unable to control the rising costs. Plans then focused on drug costs through the use of generic substitution programs, volume purchasing through mail-order distribution, benefit limitations, and drug formularies.

Health care plans now are focusing their efforts on developing programs that encourage appropriate prescribing by physicians, appropriate dispensing by pharmacists, and appropriate use by patients. Patient and physician education programs are an important part of this effort.

Some health care plans are establishing innovative financial arrangements for sharing the pharmacy benefit risk. These types of arrangements give the physician or pharmacist a financial incentive to prescribe cost-effective therapies and monitor patient utilization. Although the use of these arrangements is not yet widespread, it will continue to increase as access to prescription drug data expands and improves.

■ Underwriting and Rating

Underwriting

Prescription drug and other specialty plans generally are underwritten as a part of medical plans. The same underwriting guidelines that apply to medical plans apply to prescription drug plans. There are no pre-existing limits on pharmacy benefits.

Rating

Specialty plans typically are rated in conjunction with medical coverage for groups and individuals. As with medical coverage, the rating for specialty plans considers the age and sex of the individuals seeking coverage, since the use of services can vary based on these categories. Family size and composition (e.g., single person, family with dependents, or single parent family) also are factors in rating coverage.

In addition to considering the characteristics and utilization rates of a group or individual, the rating of specialty plan coverage is influenced by the plan benefits selected by the employer group or the insured, including:

- level of copayment;
- level of deductible;
- annual maximum benefit;
- incentives used to encourage the use of generic versus brand-name drugs;
- incentives designed to encourage insureds to use in-network pharmacies;
- availability of a mail-order program;
- incentives used to encourage the use of a mail-order program; and
- type of drug formulary used.

Regulations

Federal

The FDA regulates prescription drugs. Brand-name and generic drugs are tested by the FDA for their safety and effectiveness before being approved for use by consumers.

State

Prescription drug plan benefits must be approved by each state's insurance department. There are three areas of state regulation that particularly affect prescription drug insurance: mail-order and retail pharmacy equity; any willing pharmacy provider requirements; and mandated benefits.

Mail-Order and Retail Pharmacy Equity

Some retail pharmacies may not be able to compete with mail-order pharmacies because the latter may dispense a higher volume of drugs and, thus, be able to accept a higher level of discount. To address this concern, some states require coverage of the same number of days' supply of a prescription drug whether an insured purchases the drug through a mail-order drug program or a local pharmacy. For example, if insureds can purchase a 90-day supply of a drug through a mail-order program, they must also be able to purchase a 90-day supply of the drug through a local retail pharmacy. An alternative approach taken by some other states is to require that the same copayment apply to prescriptions filled through mail-order and retail pharmacies.

Any Willing Pharmacy Provider Requirements

Some states require that insureds be able to receive pharmacy benefits at any pharmacy that agrees to provide the same services and products for the same cost as pharmacies participating in a pharmacy provider network. This is known as any willing pharmacy provider requirement because any pharmacy willing to accept the terms and conditions of a pharmacy within the network is allowed to participate in it.

Some states may require health care plans within their states to contract with pharmacies directly or to contract only with pharmacies licensed in that state (rather than contracting with national networks).

Mandated Benefits

Many states have or are considering benefit mandates relating to prescription drugs. For example, some states require prescription drug plans to cover investigational drugs when other treatment options have been exhausted, or to cover drugs used for indications not approved by the FDA.

SPECIALTY PLANS

Vision Care Insurance

Vision care insurance provides benefits for routine preventive and corrective eye care. As a supplemental product, vision care insurance is written to complement other basic coverages. An insurer or health plan offering vision care benefits contracts with eye health professionals to provide these services at rates agreed upon by the health plan. Insureds whose health care coverage includes vision benefits usually must receive vision services from eye care professionals in the network.

One of the objectives of vision care insurance is to encourage regular or periodic eye examinations so that appropriate corrective care can be given, if needed. Vision coverage usually includes one eye exam a year and a discount on eyeglasses (both lenses and frames) or contact lenses.

The vision plan design determines the type and amounts of vision benefits available to insureds. An annual maximum benefit may apply to vision coverage.

TRICARE Supplements

TRICARE supplements are health insurance contracts with benefits that generally cover some part of the deductibles, coinsurance, and cost share amounts associated with the TRICARE program. TRICARE is the program by which the Department of Defense pays for health care delivered to members of the Uniformed Services and their families in the civilian medical community. In 1997, TRICARE replaced the Civilian Health and Medical Program of the Uniformed Services (CHAMPUS).

The supplements generally are sold as individually purchased group insurance through organizations such as the Air Force Association and the Retired Officers Association. The associations hold the

(continued)

161

group policies, and the insureds are issued individual certificates of coverage. Most associations purchase administrative services and risk assumption from third-party administrators.

TRICARE Program

The TRICARE program has three options:

- TRICARE Standard pays most of the costs of care given in civilian hospitals and by other civilian providers when a person covered under these programs cannot get care in a military hospital or clinic.
- TRICARE Extra operates like the standard program except that insureds must use a network of preferred providers.
- TRICARE Prime operates like an open-panel health maintenance organization (HMO).

Since the change from CHAMPUS to TRICARE is relatively recent, TRICARE supplement products are still being designed. Historically, the standard supplements give insureds the option of paying for inpatient and outpatient cost shares, or inpatient cost shares only. Some supplements pay for deductibles or impose their own contract deductible; others do not. Deductibles and cost shares are different for insureds in active duty than for those who are retired. Most organizations that sell supplements offer a number of these options to satisfy the needs of their customers.

Supplement coverage for TRICARE Extra is similar to the standard coverage except that benefit payments are less when an insured chooses to use a provider in the network. Insurance companies are considering additional contract design options to supplement TRICARE Extra benefits.

TRICARE Prime involves the most challenging issues of supplemental product design since many organizations are introducing first-generation coverage for these new benefits. Most policies pay outpatient and/or inpatient copayments. Enrollment fees and coverage for the point-of-service deductible usually are not covered. Cover-

(continued)

age for point-of-service cost shares ranges from no pay to full pay. As experience is gained with TRICARE Prime, future supplemental benefits may expand.

Eligibility

Persons eligible for TRICARE include certain people associated with the seven Uniformed Services: the Air Force, Army, Coast Guard, Marine Corps, National Oceanic and Atmospheric Administration, Navy, and Public Health Service. Persons covered include:

- spouses of active duty personnel;
- retirees and their spouses (up to age 65);
- reservists and their spouses (up to age 65) when called to active duty for more than 30 days;
- unmarried former spouses of active duty or retired military who were married for at least 20 years during active duty service;
- unmarried children of the eligible persons listed above who are under age 21, or under age 23 if they are full-time students.

Eligibility for the TRICARE program ends when an eligible person turns age 65 and becomes eligible for Medicare.

Summary

Specialty plans such as prescription drug insurance provide important additional coverage for Americans. Despite the rising cost of medications, prescription drug coverage is likely to continue to be an important component of health care plans. Prescription drugs generally are a more cost-effective alternative to hospitalization and other forms of medical treatment. Although challenges remain, health care plans must continue to bring drug therapy into the broad spectrum of health care to ensure optimum care. Other specialty plans such as vision care and TRICARE supplements also play an important role in providing Americans with a broader range of health care coverage.

■ Key Terms

Average wholesale price (AWP)
Brand-name drug
Copayment
Deductible
Disease state management
Dispense as written (DAW)
Dispensing fee
Drug formulary
Food and Drug Administration (FDA)
Generic drug
Generic substitution
Mail-order pharmacy
Maintenance drug
Maximum allowable cost (MAC)
Over-the-counter (OTC) drug
Pharmacy benefit manager (PBM)
Pharmacy provider network
Prescription drug
Prescription drug order
Prescription drug plan
Therapeutic substitution
TRICARE supplement
Vision care insurance

CHAPTER 8

THE SUPPLEMENTAL HEALTH INSURANCE MARKET

165 *Introduction*
168 *Factors for Success*
169 *Summary*
169 *Key Terms*

■ Introduction

Insurance carriers selling in the supplemental health insurance market today offer a rich and diverse group of products that are distributed through direct agent and broker sales, payroll deduction, telemarketing, endorsed association markets, and direct response sales. These products and distribution techniques are designed to meet the various needs of the consumer.

The demand for supplemental health insurance is likely to increase as the gaps in individual and group medical expense coverage continue to increase. According to a Louis A. Harris and Associates survey conducted in 1996 for the Center for Studying Health System Change, 64 percent of the 5,111 respondents reported that their out-of-pocket costs increased over the past three years. Twenty-six percent said their family health care costs are somewhat or completely out of control. Fully 9 of 10 respondents expect their out-of-pocket costs to rise.[23 p.194]

While the demand for supplemental health insurance products is likely to increase, the number of carriers in the market may be decreasing based on two factors:

- the mergers of supplemental companies in competing businesses; and
- traditional carriers acquiring blocks of business to avoid the expense and time of developing their own new products.

Market and Product Changes

Supplemental health insurance products are designed to fill the gaps in basic health insurance coverage to provide broader protection against risks. The popularity of supplemental health insurance products is expected to continue to grow and insurance carriers will continue to develop new products to meet consumer demand. Competition in the supplemental market will cause most insurers to do something to make their product unique, whether through product design, pricing, customer service, or some other value-added feature.

Managed Care

Health maintenance organizations (HMOs) and other managed care plans have grown in response to market pressures to reduce health care costs and manage demand for health care services. There are many levels of managed care medical expense insurance products in the market and many of them contain the same uncovered expenses as traditional indemnity plans. The gaps could be even larger if enrollees elect to use health care services that are out of a plan's network.

Consumer awareness that managed care plans bear the same financial responsibility for certain uncovered expenses is increasing. As a result of this enhanced awareness, more people are likely to decide they need supplemental health insurance coverage.

Cost Management

Cost management techniques, whether used by HMOs or indemnity plans, also could lead to an increase in supplemental health insurance sales. For example, as a cost saving technique, increasingly shorter hospital stays have become the norm. This development has promoted the need for hospital indemnity insurance, a leading supplemental product.

Another factor that has provided tremendous growth opportunities is that many employers feel they have reached their limit in how much they can cut back on benefits and shift costs to their employees. Already many employers offer less comprehensive plans, which means more gaps for supplemental products to fill. Employers are turning their defined benefit plans into defined contribution plans so that employees can choose which benefits they want. This holds down the costs for employers while increasing the range of supplemental insurance products for employees.

Medicare Supplement

Medicare supplement plans have been a strong part of the supplemental market, but insurers may see a stagnating market here—or even a reduction in sales—in the future. Part of this trend is due to regulation and part to consumer choice (moving from indemnity coverage to Medicare HMOs).

With the new Medicare+Choice, the Medicare supplement market will face increased challenges from HMOs, as more people over age 65 enroll in these managed care plans to save money. Health insurers will face tremendous pressure trying to balance higher utilization of health services in a market that expects quality products, affordable prices, and above average customer service.

Federal and State Regulations

Traditionally, health insurance has been regulated at the state level, but in recent years the federal government has broadened its involvement in insurance issues. Currently, no federal regulation prohibits the sale of supplemental health insurance products to consumers.

The National Association of Insurance Commissioners (NAIC) will be reviewing several issues related to supplemental insurance products. These issues include: loss ratios, disclosure, minimum benefits, and risk classification—issues that could cause supplemental insurers to make changes in their products, premiums, and marketing strategies.

Data Collection

Advances in data collection and management will likely give supplemental health insurers new marketing methods. For example, with the availability of sophisticated databases of potential customers, insurers will be in a better position to know who are candidates for mass marketing. Insurers can study the buying habits of their customers and know which individuals previously bought products and whether they are likely to purchase products in the future.

Distribution

In addition to product changes, the supplemental health insurance market will encounter changes in distribution methods. Some of these include:

- *Payroll deduction.* Employers will continue to offer their employees voluntary supplemental health insurance plans through payroll deduction because it allows them to provide a comprehensive benefit package without the costs associated with employer-paid plans.
- *Banks.* As banks expand into the insurance market, consumers will become more aware of the wide range of supplemental health products, which will lead to further expansion of the market for insurers. Many insurers and banks are setting up partnership arrangements to take advantage of each other's specialties, while consolidating larger customer bases for both industries.
- *Internet.* The Internet is just beginning to be used for sales of supplemental products. As more people go on-line and data are collected regarding who they are and how they make buying decisions, the Internet will expand to reach these customers and meet their needs.

Factors for Success

There is no one model for success, but a general business principle for successful companies is to be alert to and mindful of changes in the marketplace. The following factors provide some of the important elements of a successful marketing effort:

- *Affordable products.* No matter how good an insurance product is, it must be purchased to be of benefit to the insured.
- *Consumer awareness.* Make sure that potential customers realize the need for your product.
- *Know your market.* Supplemental products must be designed and marketed to fill the needs of new and potential insureds. Insurers must target the right product to the right customers.

- *Distribution.* Successful companies match their customers to the appropriate distribution method.
- *Customer service.* Customers want personal attention in meeting their supplemental health insurance needs and companies must learn how to provide service in a cost-effective manner.
- *Access customer data.* Finding the right data enhances the sales process and helps improve profitability.
- *Flexibility.* A company's customer needs change over time, and successful insurers change to meet the needs of new and different customers.
- *Develop critical mass.* Successful companies will continually develop or acquire new products or blocks of coverage that other companies have but no longer want.
- *Think globally.* The market for supplemental products is growing beyond the United States; opportunities currently exist in Japan and Canada.

Summary

The supplemental health insurance market is poised to face a viable and changing marketplace. Companies that provide affordable products that meet the need of their customers, will continue to grow and dominate the market.

Key Terms

Banks
Defined contribution
Distribution methods
Employee benefits
Health maintenance organizations (HMOs)
Internet
Loss ratio
Managed care
Medicare supplement
National Association of Insurance Commissioners (NAIC)
Payroll deduction
Risk classification
Supplemental health insurance

Appendix A

INDIVIDUAL ACCIDENT AND SICKNESS INSURANCE MINIMUM STANDARDS ACT

(Model Regulation Service—October 1995)

From the NAIC *Model Laws, Regulations and Guidelines.* Reprinted with permission of the National Association of Insurance Commissioners.

Table of Contents

Section 1.	Purpose
Section 2.	Definitions
Section 3.	Standards for Policy Provisions
Section 4.	Minimum Standards for Benefits
Section 5.	Disclosure Requirements
Section 6.	Preexisting Conditions
Section 7.	Administrative Procedures

Section 1. Purpose

The purpose of this Act shall be to provide reasonable standardization and simplification of terms and coverages of individual accident and sickness insurance policies and subscriber contracts of nonprofit hospital, medical and dental service associations to facilitate public understanding and comparison, to eliminate provisions contained in individual accident and sickness insurance policies and subscriber contracts of nonprofit hospital, medical and dental service associations which may be misleading or unreasonably confusing in connection either with the purchase of such coverages or with the settlement of claims, and to provide for full disclosure in the sale of accident and sickness coverages. This Act shall not apply to insurance policies and subscriber contracts subject to the [Medicare Supplement Insurance Minimum Standards Act].

Section 2. Definitions

A. "Accident and sickness insurance" means insurance written under [insert here the section of law authorizing accident and sickness insurance], other than credit accident and sickness insurance, and coverages written under [insert here the section of law authorizing nonprofit hospital, medical and dental service associations]. For purposes of this Act, nonprofit hospital, medical and dental service associations shall be deemed to be engaged in the business of insurance.

B. "Form" means policies, contracts, riders, endorsements and applications as provided in [cite section of state law regarding the filing and approval of individual accident and sickness insurance policy forms and subscriber contracts of nonprofit hospital, medical and dental service associations].

Drafting Note: This definition may be unnecessary if the term "form" is appropriately defined elsewhere, but it may be considered helpful to include it here with an appropriate cross-reference.

C. "Policy" means the entire contract between the insurer and the insured, including the policy riders, endorsements and the application, if attached; and also includes subscriber contracts issued by nonprofit hospital, medical and dental service associations.

Section 3. Standards for Policy Provisions

A. The commissioner shall issue regulations to establish specific standards, including standards of full and fair disclosure, that set forth the manner, content and required disclosure for the sale of individual policies of accident and sickness insurance and subscriber contracts of nonprofit hospital, medical and dental service associations, other than conversion policies issued pursuant to a contractual conversion privilege under a group or individual policy of accident and sickness insurance, when such group or individual contract contains provisions which are inconsistent with the requirements of this Act or any regulation issued pursuant to the Act, or to policies being issued to employees or members being added to franchise plans in existence on the effective date of this Act or any regulation issued pursuant to the Act, which shall be in addition to and in accordance with applicable laws of this State, including the [insert applicable statutory reference to Uniform Individual Accident and Sickness Policy Provisions Law], which may cover but shall not be limited to:

  (1)   Terms of renewability;

  (2)   Initial and subsequent conditions of eligibility;

  (3)   Nonduplication of coverage provisions;

  (4)   Coverage of dependents;

  (5)   Preexisting conditions;

  (6)   Termination of insurance;

  (7)   Probationary periods;

  (8)   Limitations;

  (9)   Exceptions;

  (10) Reductions;

  (11) Elimination periods;

  (12) Requirements for replacement;

  (13) Recurrent conditions; and

  (14) The definition of terms including but not limited to the following: hospital, accident, sickness, injury, physician, accidental means, total disability, partial disability, nervous disorder, guaranteed renewable and noncancellable.

Drafting Note: This section authorizes the commissioner to establish specific standards for policy provisions that will facilitate public understanding of the provisions. The section does not alter the requirements of the Uniform Individual Accident and Sickness Policy Provisions Law (UPPL) or other specifically applicable state laws dealing with individual policy provisions. Regulations adopted under this section should be consistent with the UPPL and other applicable state laws relating to the subject matter. The phrase "including standards of full and fair disclosure" provides the commissioner authority to establish standards which are not only technically accurate and in clear language but which, in addition, are stated in a manner to insure that their significance is fully understood.

B. The commissioner may issue regulations that specify prohibited policies or policy provisions not otherwise specifically authorized by statute which in the opinion of the commissioner are unjust, unfair, or unfairly discriminatory to the policyholder, any person insured under the policy, or a beneficiary.

Section 4. Minimum Standards for Benefits

A. The commissioner shall issue regulations to establish minimum standards for benefits under each of the following categories of coverage in individual policies, other than conversion policies issued pursuant to a contractual conversion privilege under a group or individual policy, when the group or individual contract contains provisions which are inconsistent with the requirements of this Act or any regulation issued pursuant to the Act or to policies being issued to employees or members being added to franchise plans in existence on the effective date of this Act or any regulation issued pursuant to the Act, of accident and sickness insurance and subscriber contracts of nonprofit hospital, medical and dental service associations:

   (1) Basic hospital expense coverage;

   (2) Basic medical-surgical expense coverage;

   (3) Hospital confinement indemnity coverage;

   (4) Major medical expense coverage;

   (5) Disability income protection coverage;

   (6) Accident only coverage;

   (7) Specified disease or specified accident coverage; and

   (8) Limited benefit health coverage.

Drafting Note: "Specified disease or specified accident coverage" refers to a coverage which contains unusual exclusions, limitations, reductions, or conditions of such a restrictive nature that the payments of benefits under such a policy or contract are limited in frequency or in amounts. An example of such a specified disease or specified accident coverage would be a cancer only hospital indemnity policy or an automobile accident only policy. Such coverages are referred to as "limited policies" in the NAIC Official Guide for the Filing and Approval of Accident and Health Contracts and the 1965 statement of Underwriting Practices of Individual Accident and Health Policies (1966 *Proceedings of the NAIC* I, pages 132-134).

B. Nothing in this section shall preclude the issuance of any policy or contract which combines two (2) or more of the categories of coverage enumerated in Paragraphs (1) through (8) of Subsection A.

Drafting Note: This subsection does not restrict reasonable combinations of those coverages in Paragraphs (1) through (8). For example, accident only coverage may be issued in conjunction with other categories. However, the section does not permit the combination of specified disease or specified accident coverages with other categories of coverage unless specifically permitted by any regulation adopted pursuant to this Act.

C. No policy or contract shall be delivered or issued for delivery in this state which does not meet the prescribed minimum standards for the categories of coverage listed in Paragraphs (1) through (8) of Subsection A or does not meet the requirements set forth in [cite applicable section of state law authorizing the commissioner to disapprove individual policy forms if the benefits provided therein are unreasonable in relation to the premium charged].

D. The commissioner shall prescribe the method of identification of policies and contracts based upon coverages provided.

Section 5. Disclosure Requirements

A. In order to provide for full and fair disclosure in the sale of individual accident and sickness insurance policies or subscriber contracts of a non-profit hospital, medical or dental service association, no policy or contract shall be delivered or issued for delivery in this state unless the outline of coverage described in Subsection B either accompanies the policy or is delivered to the applicant at the time application is made and an acknowledgement of receipt or certificate of delivery of the outline is provided the insurer. In the event the policy is issued on a basis other than that applied for, the outline of coverage properly describing the policy or contract must accompany the policy or contract when it is not the policy or contract for which application was made.

B. The commissioner shall prescribe the format and content of the outline of coverage required by Subsection A. "Format" means style, arrangement and overall appearance, including such items as the size, color and prominence of type and the arrangement of text and captions. The outline of coverage shall include:

(1) A statement identifying the applicable category or categories of coverage provided by the policy or contract as prescribed in Section 4 of this Act;

(2) A description of the principal benefits and coverage provided in the policy or contract;

(3) A statement of the exceptions, reductions and limitations contained in the policy or contract;

(4) A statement of the renewal provisions including any reservation by the insurer of nonprofit hospital, medical or dental service association of a right to change premiums; and

(5) A statement that the outline is a summary of the policy or contract issued or applied for and that the policy or contract should be consulted to determine governing contractual provisions.

Drafting Note: Any possible conflict with Section 3A(1) of the Uniform Individual Accident and Sickness Policy Provisions Law can be avoided by enclosing and not attaching the outline at the time of policy or contract delivery.

Section 6. Preexisting Conditions

A. [Those jurisdictions which have not already done so should amend Section 3A(2)(a) and (b), the "Time Limits on Certain Defenses" and "Incontestable" provisions of the Uniform Individual Accident and Sickness Policy Provisions Act to reduce the permissible time limit of preexisting conditions from three years to not more than two years].

B. Notwithstanding the provisions of [insert applicable statutory reference to Section 3A(2)(b) of the Uniform Individual Accident and Sickness Policy Provisions Law], if an insurer or a nonprofit hospital, medical or dental service association elects to use a simplified application form, with or without a question as to the applicant's health at the time of application, but without any questions concerning the insured's health history or medical treatment history, the policy must cover any loss occurring after twelve (12) months from any preexisting condition not specifically excluded from coverage by terms of the policy, and, except as so provided, the policy or contract shall not include wording that would permit a defense based upon preexisting conditions.

Drafting Note: Subsection B is based upon the 1965 NAIC statement of Underwriting Practices of Individual Accident and Health Policies (1966 *Proceedings of the NAIC* I, pages 132-134).

C. Notwithstanding the provisions of Subsections A or B and the provisions of [insert applicable statutory reference to Section 3A(2)(b) of the Uniform Individual Accident and Sickness Policy Provisions Law] an insurer or a nonprofit hospital, medical or dental service association which issues a specified disease policy, regardless of whether such policy is issued on the basis of a detailed application form, a simplified application form or an enrollment form, may not deny a claim for any covered loss that begins after the policy has been in force for at least six (6) months, unless such loss results from a preexisting condition which first manifests itself within six (6) months prior to the effective date of the policy or contract or was diagnosed by a physician at any time prior to such a date. Except for rescission for misrepresentation, no other defenses based upon preexisting conditions are permitted.

Section 7. Administrative Procedures

Regulations promulgated pursuant to this Act shall be subject to notice and hearing pursuant to [cite section of law relating to the adoption and promulgation of rules and regulations or state Administrative Procedures Act].

General Drafting Notes: In preparing the Act for introduction in a legislative body:

1. The term "commissioner" should be replaced with "director" or "superintendent" where appropriate under state law.
2. The phrase "accident and sickness" should be replaced by "accident and disability," "accident and health," or such other phrases as may be appropriate under state law.
3. The phrase "nonprofit hospital, medical and dental service associations" should be replaced with terms conforming to state statutes.
4. The term "regulation" should be replaced by the terms "rules and regulations" or "rules" where appropriate under state law.
5. The term "individual" as used in this Act corresponds to its use in the Uniform Individual Accident and Sickness Policy Provisions Law, thus extending the coverage of the Act to "family" policies.
6. State laws authorizing nonprofit hospital, medical, and dental service associations may require the modification of the model Act in order to make it applicable to such organizations.

Legislative History (all references are to the Proceedings of the NAIC).

1974 Proc. I 12, 14, 405, 413, 414-418 (adopted).
1977 Proc. I 26, 28, 49-53, 317, 325 (amended and reprinted).
1979 Proc. I 44, 47, 373, 385, 394-396 (amended).
1980 Proc. II 22, 26, 588, 591, 594, 634 (amended).
1989 Proc. II 13, 23-24, 467-468, 518-519, 544-548 (amended to remove references to Medicare supplement insurance).

Appendix B

MODEL REGULATION TO IMPLEMENT THE INDIVIDUAL ACCIDENT AND SICKNESS INSURANCE MINIMUM STANDARDS ACT

(Model Regulation Service—July 1997)

From the NAIC *Model Laws, Regulations and Guidelines*. Reprinted with permission of the National Association of Insurance Commissioners.

Table of Contents

Section 1.	Purpose
Section 2.	Authority
Section 3.	Applicability and Scope
Section 4.	Effective Date
Section 5.	Policy Definitions
Section 6.	Prohibited Policy Provisions
Section 7.	Accident and Sickness Minimum Standards for Benefits
Section 8.	Required Disclosure Provisions
Section 9.	Requirements for Replacement
Section 10.	Separability

Section 1.   Purpose

The purpose of this regulation is to implement [cite section of law which sets forth the NAIC Individual Accident and Sickness Insurance Minimum Standards Act] so as to provide reasonable standardization and simplification of terms and coverages of individual accident and sickness insurance policies and individual subscriber contracts of hospital, medical and dental service corporations in order to facilitate public understanding and comparison and to eliminate provisions contained in individual accident and sickness insurance policies and individual subscriber contracts of hospital, medical and dental service corporations which may be misleading or confusing in connection either with the purchase of such coverages or with the settlement of claims, and to provide for full disclosure in the sale of such coverages.

Section 2.   Authority

This regulation is issued pursuant to the authority vested in the commissioner under [cite appropriate section of law enacting NAIC Individual Accident and Sickness Insurance Minimum Standards Act and any other appropriate section of law regarding authority of commissioner to issue or promulgate rules and regulations].

SUPPLEMENTAL HEALTH INSURANCE

Section 3. Applicability and Scope

This regulation shall apply to all individual accident and sickness insurance policies and subscriber contracts of hospital, medical and dental service corporations delivered or issued for delivery in this state on and after the effective date hereof, except it shall not apply to:

- A. Individual policies or contracts issued pursuant to a conversion privilege under a policy or contract of group or individual insurance when such group or individual policy or contract includes provisions which are inconsistent with the requirements of this regulation;

- B. Policies being issued to employees or members as additions to franchise plans in existence on the effective date of this regulation;

- C. Medicare supplement policies subject to [cite rule implementing the Medicare Supplement Insurance Minimum Standards Regulation];

- D. Long-term care insurance policies subject to [cite rule implementing the Long-Term Care Insurance Act].

The requirements contained in this regulation shall be in addition to any other applicable regulations previously adopted.

Section 4. Effective Date

This regulation shall be effective on [insert a date not less than 120 days after the date of adoption or promulgation of the regulation] and shall be applicable to all individual accident and sickness insurance policies and nonprofit hospital, medical and dental service contracts delivered or issued for delivery in this state on and after such date which are not specifically exempt from this regulation.

Section 5. Policy Definitions

Except as provided hereafter, no individual accident or sickness insurance policy or hospital, medical or dental service corporation subscriber contract delivered or issued for delivery to any person in this state and to which this regulation applies shall contain definitions respecting the matters set forth below unless such definitions comply with the requirements of this section.

- A. "One period of confinement" means consecutive days of in-hospital service received as an in-patient, or successive confinements when discharge from and readmission to the hospital occurs within a period of time not more than ninety (90) days or three times the maximum number of days of in-hospital coverage provided by the policy to a maximum of 180 days.

- B. "Hospital" may be defined in relation to its status, facilities and available services or to reflect its accreditation by the Joint Commission on Accreditation of Hospitals.

(1) The definition of the term "hospital" shall not be more restrictive than one requiring that the hospital:

    (a) Be an institution operated pursuant to law; and

    (b) Be primarily and continuously engaged in providing or operating; either on its premises or in facilities available to the hospital on a prearranged basis and under the supervision of a staff of duly licensed physicians; medical, diagnostic and major surgical facilities for the medical care and treatment of sick or injured persons on an in-patient basis for which a charge is made; and

    (c) Provide twenty-four-hour nursing service by or under the supervision of registered graduate professional nurses (R.N.s).

(2) The definition of the term "hospital" may state that such term shall not be inclusive of:

    (a) Convalescent homes, convalescent, rest, or nursing facilities; or

    (b) Facilities primarily affording custodial, educational or rehabilitory care; or

    (c) Facilities for the aged, drug addicts or alcoholics; or

    (d) Any military or veterans hospital or soldiers home or any hospital contracted for or operated by any national government or agency thereof for the treatment of members or ex-members of the armed forces, except for services rendered on an emergency basis where a legal liability exists for charges made to the individual for such services.

Drafting Note: The laws of the several states relating to the type of hospital facilities recognized in health insurance policies are not uniform. References to individual state law may be required in structuring this definition of this regulation.

    C. "Convalescent Nursing Home," "Extended Care Facility," or "Skilled Nursing Facility" shall be defined in relation to its status, facilities, and available services.

    (1) A definition of such home or facility shall not be more restrictive than one requiring that it:

        (a) Be operated pursuant to law;

        (b) Be approved for payment of Medicare benefits or be qualified to receive such approval, if so requested;

SUPPLEMENTAL HEALTH INSURANCE

(c) Be primarily engaged in providing, in addition to room and board accommodations, skilled nursing care under the supervision of a duly licensed physician;

(d) Provide continuous twenty-four-hour-a-day nursing service by or under the supervision of a registered graduate professional nurse (R.N.); and

(e) Maintains a daily medical record of each patient.

(2) The definition of such home or facility may provide that such term shall not be inclusive of:

(a) Any home, facility or part thereof used primarily for rest;

(b) A home or facility for the aged or for the care of drug addicts or alcoholics; or

(c) A home or facility primarily used for the care and treatment of mental diseases, or disorders, or custodial or educational care.

Drafting Note: The laws of the several states relating to nursing and extended care facilities recognized in health insurance policies are not uniform. Reference to the individual state law may be required in structuring this definition of this regulation.

D. "Accident," "Accidental Injury," "Accidental Means" shall be defined to employ "result" language and shall not include words which establish an accidental means test or use words such as "external, violent, visible wounds" or similar words of description or characterization.

The definition shall not be more restrictive than the following: Injury or injuries, for which benefits are provided, means accidental bodily injury sustained by the insured person which are the direct cause, independent of disease or bodily infirmity or any other cause and occur while the insurance is in force.

Such definition may provide that injuries shall not include injuries for which benefits are provided under workmen's compensation, employer's liability or similar law, motor vehicle no-fault plan, unless prohibited by law, or injuries occurring while the insured person is engaged in any activity pertaining to any trade, business, employment, or occupation for wage or profit.

E. "Sickness" shall not be defined to be more restrictive than the following: Sickness means sickness or disease of an insured person which first manifests itself after the effective date of insurance and while the insurance is in force. A definition of sickness may provide for a probationary period which will not exceed thirty (30) days from the effective date of the coverage of the insured person. The definition may be further modified to exclude sickness or disease for which benefits are provided under any workman's compensation, occupational disease, employer's liability or similar law.

F. "Preexisting condition" shall not be defined to be more restrictive than the following: Preexisting condition means the existence of symptoms which would cause an ordinarily prudent person to seek diagnosis, care or treatment within a five (5) year period preceding the effective date of the coverage of the insured person or a condition for which medical advice or treatment was recommended by a physician or received from a physician within a five (5) year period preceding the effective date of the coverage of the insured person.

Drafting Note: This definition does not prohibit an insurer, using an application form designed to elicit the complete health history of a prospective insured and on the basis of the answers on that application, from underwriting in accordance with that insurer's established standards. It is assumed that an insurer that elicits a complete health history of a prospective insured will act on the information and if the review of the health history results in a decision to exclude a condition, the policy will be endorsed or amended by including the specific exclusion. This same requirement of notice to the prospective insured of the specific exclusion will also apply to insurers which elect to use simplified application forms containing questions relating to the prospective insured's health.

This definition does, however, prohibit an insurer that elects to use a simplified application, with or without a question as to the applicant's health at the time of application, from reducing or denying a claim on the basis of the existence of a preexisting condition that is defined more restrictively than above.

G. "Physician" may be defined by including words such as "duly qualified physician" or "duly licensed physician." The use of such terms requires an insurer to recognize and to accept, to the extent of its obligation under the contract, all providers of medical care and treatment when such services are within the scope of the provider's licensed authority and are provided pursuant to applicable laws.

Note: The laws of the several states relating to the type of practitioners services recognized in health insurance policies are not uniform. References to the individual state law may be required in structuring this definition of this regulation.

H. "Nurses" may be defined so that the description of nurse is restricted to a type of nurse, such as registered graduate professional nurse (R.N.), a licensed practical nurse (L.P.N.), or a licensed vocational nurse (L.V.N). If the words "nurse," "trained nurse" or "registered nurse" are used without specific instruction, then the use of such terms requires the insurer to recognize the services of any individual who qualifies under such terminology in accordance with the applicable statutes or administrative rules of the licensing or registry board of the state.

I. "Total Disability"

- (1) A general definition of total disability cannot be more restrictive than one requiring that the individual who is totally disabled not be engaged in any employment or occupation for which he is or becomes qualified by reason of education, training or experience; and not in fact engaged in any employment or occupation for wage or profit.

- (2) Total disability may be defined in relation to the inability of the person to perform duties but may not be based solely upon an individual's inability to:

    - (a) Perform "any occupation whatsoever," "any occupational duty," or "any and every duty of his occupation," or

    - (b) Engage in any training or rehabilitation program.

- (3) An insurer may specify the requirement of the complete inability of the person to perform all of the substantial and material duties of his regular occupation or words of similar import. An insurer may require care by a physician (other than the insured or a member of the insured's immediate family).

J. "Partial Disability" shall be defined in relation to the individual's inability to perform one or more but not all of the "major," "important" or "essential" duties of employment or occupation or may be related to a percentage of time worked or to a specified number of hours or to compensation. Where a policy provides total disability benefits and partial disability benefits, only one elimination period may be required.

K. "Residual Disability" shall be defined in relation to the individual's reduction in earnings and may be related either to the inability to perform some part of the "major," "important" or "essential duties" of employment or occupation, or to the inability to perform all usual business duties for as long as is usually required. A policy which provides for residual disability benefits may require a qualification period, during which the insured must be continuously totally disabled before residual disability benefits are payable. The qualification period for residual benefits may be longer than the elimination period for total disability. In lieu of the term "residual disability," the insurer may use "proportionate disability" or other term of similar import which in the opinion of the commissioner adequately and fairly describes the benefit.

L. "Medicare" shall be substantially defined as "The Health Insurance for the Aged Act, Title XVIII of the Social Security Amendments of 1965 as Then Constituted or Later Amended," or "Title I, Part I of Public Laws 89-97, as Enacted by the Eighty-Ninth Congress of the United States of America and popularly known as

APPENDIX B

the Health Insurance for the Aged Act," as then constituted and any later amendments or substitutes thereof" or words of similar import.

M. "Mental or Nervous Disorder" shall not be defined more restrictively than a definition including neurosis, psychoneurosis, psychosis, or mental or emotional disease or disorder of any kind.

Section 6. Prohibited Policy Provisions

A. Except as provided in Section 5E, no policy shall contain provisions establishing a probationary or waiting period during which no coverage is provided under the policy, subject to the further exception that a policy may specify a probationary or waiting period not to exceed six (6) months for specified diseases or conditions and losses resulting therefrom for hernia, disorder of reproduction organs, varicose veins, adenoids, appendix and tonsils. However, the permissible six (6) months exception shall not be applicable where such specified diseases or conditions are treated on an emergency basis. Accident policies shall not contain probationary or waiting periods.

B. No policy or rider for additional coverage may be issued as a dividend unless an equivalent cash payment is offered to the policyholder as an alternative to such dividend policy or rider. No such dividend policy or rider shall be issued for an initial term of less than six (6) months.

The initial renewal subsequent to the issuance of any policy or rider as a dividend shall clearly disclose that the policyholder is renewing the coverage that was provided as a dividend for the previous term and that such renewal is optional with the policyholder.

C. No policy shall exclude coverage for a loss due to a preexisting condition for a period greater than twelve (12) months following policy issue where the application for such insurance does not seek disclosure of prior illness, disease or physical conditions or prior medical care and treatment and such preexisting condition is not specifically excluded by the terms of the policy.

Drafting Note: Where the jurisdiction has enacted the 1973 NAIC Individual Accident and Sickness Insurance Minimum Standard Act this provision is unnecessary.

D. A disability income policy may contain a "return of premium" or "cash value benefit" so long as: (1) such return of premium or cash value benefit is not reduced by an amount greater than the aggregate of any claims paid under the policy; and (2) the insurer demonstrates that the reserve basis for such policies is adequate. No other policy shall provide a return of premium or cash value benefit, except return of unearned premium upon termination or suspension of coverage, retroactive waiver of premium paid during disability, payment of dividends on participating policies, or experience rating refunds.

Drafting Note: This provision is optional and the desirability of its use should be reviewed by the individual states.

E. Policies providing hospital confinement indemnity coverage shall not contain provisions excluding coverage because of confinement in a hospital operated by the federal government.

F. No policy shall limit or exclude coverage by type of illness, accident, treatment or medical condition, except as follows:

(1) Preexisting conditions or diseases, except for congenital anomalies of a covered dependent child;

(2) Mental or emotional disorders, alcoholism and drug addition;

(3) Pregnancy, except for complications of pregnancy, other than for policies defined in Section 7F of this regulation;

(4) Illness, treatment or medical condition arising out of:

(a) War or act of war (whether declared or undeclared); participation in a felony, riot or insurrections; service in the armed forces or units auxiliary thereto,

(b) Suicide (sane or insane), attempted suicide or intentionally self-inflicted injury,

(c) Aviation,

(d) With respect to short-term nonrenewable policies, interscholastic sports;

(5) Cosmetic surgery, except that "cosmetic surgery" shall not include reconstructive surgery when such service is incidental to or follows surgery resulting from trauma, infection or other diseases of the involved part, and reconstructive surgery because of congenital disease or anomaly of a covered dependent child which has resulted in a functional defect;

(6) Foot care in connection with corns, calluses, flat feet, fallen arches, weak feet, chronic foot strain, or symptomatic complaints of the feet;

(7) Care in connection with the detection and correction by manual or mechanical means of structural imbalance, distortion, or subluxation in the human body for purposes of removing nerve interference and the effects thereof, where such interference is the result of or related to distortion, misalignment or subluxation of, or in the vertebral column;

EDITOR'S NOTE: When adopting this model, states should examine any existing "freedom of choice" statutes which require reimbursement of treatment provided by chiropractors, and make adjustments if needed.

APPENDIX B

    (8)   Treatment provided in a government hospital; benefits provided under Medicare or other governmental program (except Medicaid), any state or federal workmen's compensation, employers liability or occupational disease law, or any motor vehicle no-fault law; services rendered by employees of hospitals, laboratories or other institutions; services performed by a member of the covered person's immediate family; and services for which no charge is normally made in the absence of insurance.

    (9)   Dental care or treatment;

    (10)   Eye glasses, hearing aids and examination for the prescription or fitting thereof;

    (11)   Rest cures, custodial care, transportation and routine physical examinations;

    (12)   Territorial limitations.

Drafting Note: Some of the exclusions set forth in this provision may be unnecessary or in conflict with existing state legislation and, thus, should be deleted.

    G.   This regulation shall not impair or limit the use of waivers to exclude, limit or reduce coverage or benefits for specifically named or described preexisting diseases, physical condition or extra hazardous activity. Where waivers are required as a condition of issuance, renewal or reinstatement, signed acceptance by the insured is required unless on initial issuance the full text of the waiver is contained either on the first page or specification page.

    H.   Policy provisions precluded in this section shall not be construed as a limitation on the authority of the commissioner to disapprove other policy provisions in accordance with [cite Section 3B of the Individual Accident and Sickness Insurance Minimum Standards Act] which in the opinion of the commissioner are unjust, unfair, or unfairly discriminatory to the policyholders, beneficiary or any person insured under the policy.

Section 7.   Accident and Sickness Minimum Standards for Benefits

The following minimum standards for benefits are prescribed for the categories of coverage noted in the following subsections. No individual policy of accident and sickness insurance or nonprofit hospital, medical or dental service corporation contract shall be delivered or issued for delivery in this state which does not meet the required minimum standards for the specified categories unless the commissioner finds that such policies or contracts are approvable as limited benefit health insurance and the outline of coverage complies with the appropriate outline in Section 8L of this regulation.

Nothing in this section shall preclude the issuance of any policy or contract combining two or more categories set forth in [cite Section 4A and B of the Model Act].

SUPPLEMENTAL HEALTH INSURANCE

A. General Rules

(1) A "noncancellable," "guaranteed renewable," or "noncancellable and guaranteed renewable" policy shall not provide for termination of coverage of the spouse solely because of the occurrence of an event specified for termination of coverage of the insured, other than nonpayment of premium. The policy shall provide that in the event of the insured's death, the spouse of the insured, if covered under the policy, shall become the insured.

(2) The terms "noncancellable," "guaranteed renewable," or "noncancellable and guaranteed renewable" shall not be used without further explanatory language in accordance with the disclosure requirements of Section 8A(1). The terms "noncancellable" or "noncancellable and guaranteed renewable" may be used only in a policy which the insured has the right to continue in force by the timely payment of premiums set forth in the policy until the age of sixty-five (65) or to eligibility for Medicare, during which period the insurer has no right to make unilaterally any change in any provision of the policy while the policy is in force: Provided however, any accident and health or accident-only policy which provides for periodic payments, weekly or monthly, for a specified period during the continuance of disability resulting from accident or sickness may provide that the insured has the right to continue the policy only to age sixty (60) if, at age sixty (60), the insured has the right to continue the policy in force at least to age sixty-five (65) while actively or regularly employed. Except as provided above, the term "guaranteed renewable" may be used only in a policy which the insured has the right to continue in force by the timely payment of premiums until the age of sixty-five (65) or to eligibility for Medicare, during which period the insurer has no right to make unilaterally any change in any provision of the policy while the policy is in force, except that the insurer may make changes in premium rates by classes: Provided however, any accident and health or accident-only policy which provides for periodic payments, weekly or monthly, for a specified period during the continuance of disability resulting from accident or sickness may provide that the insured has the right to continue the policy only to age sixty (60) if, at age sixty (60), the insured has the right to continue the policy in force at least to age sixty-five (65) while actively and regularly employed.

(3) In a family policy covering both husband and wife the age of the younger spouse must be used as the basis for meeting the age and durational requirements of the definitions of "noncancellable" or "guaranteed renewable." However, this requirement shall not prevent termination of coverage of the older spouse upon attainment of the stated age limit (e.g., age 65) so long as the policy may be continued in force as to the younger spouse to the age or for the durational period as specified in said definition.

APPENDIX B

(4) When accidental death and dismemberment coverage is part of the insurance coverage offered under the contract, the insured shall have the option to include all insureds under such coverage and not just the principal insured.

(5) If a policy contains a status-type military service exclusion or a provision which suspends coverage during military service, the policy shall provide, upon receipt of written request, for refund of premiums as applicable to such person on a pro rata basis.

(6) In the event the insurer cancels or refuses to renew, policies providing pregnancy benefits shall provide for an extension of benefits as to pregnancy commencing while the policy is in force and for which benefits would have been payable had the policy remained in force.

(7) Policies providing convalescent or extended care benefits following hospitalization shall not condition such benefits upon admission to the convalescent or extended care facility within a period of less than fourteen (14) days after discharge from the hospital.

(8) Family coverage shall continue for any dependent child who is incapable of self-sustaining employment due to mental retardation or physical handicap on the date that such child's coverage would otherwise terminate under the policy due to the attainment of a specified age limit for children and is chiefly dependent on the insured for support and maintenance. The policy may require than within thirty-one (31) days of such date the company receive due proof of such incapacity in order for the insured to elect to continue the policy in force with respect to such child, or that a separate converted policy be issued at the option of the insured or policyholder.

(9) Any policy providing coverage for the recipient in a transplant operation shall also provide reimbursement of any medical expenses of a live donor to the extent that benefits remain and are available under the recipient's policy, after benefits for the recipient's own expenses have been paid.

(10) A policy may contain a provision relating to recurrent disabilities; provided however, that no such provision shall specify that a recurrent disability be separated by a period greater than six (6) months.

(11) Accidental death and dismemberment benefits shall be payable if the loss occurs within ninety (90) days from the date of the accident, irrespective of total disability. Disability income benefits, if provided, shall not require the loss to commence less than thirty (30) days after the date of accident, nor shall any policy which the insurer cancels or refuses to renew require that it be in force at the time disability commences if the accident occurred while the policy was in force.

(12) Specific dismemberment benefits shall not be in lieu of other benefits unless the specific benefit equals or exceeds the other benefits.

(13) Any accident-only policy providing benefits which vary according to the type of accidental cause shall prominently set forth in the outline of coverage the circumstances under which benefits are payable which are lesser than the maximum amount payable under the policy.

(14) Termination of the policy shall be without prejudice ~~of~~ to any continuous loss which commenced while the policy was in force, but the extension of benefits beyond the period the policy was in force may be predicated upon the continuous total disability of the insured, limited to the duration of the policy benefit period, if any, or payment of the maximum benefits.

B. Basic Hospital Expense Coverage

"Basic Hospital Expense Coverage" is a policy of accident and sickness insurance which provides coverage for a period of not less than thirty-one (31) days during any continuous hospital confinement for each person insured under the policy, for expense incurred for necessary treatment and services rendered as a result of accident or sickness for at least the following:

(1) Daily hospital room and board in an amount not less than the lesser of (a) [80%] of the charges for semiprivate room accommodations or (b) [$30] per day;

Drafting Note: The material in brackets is variable so that a commissioner may determine the level of daily room and board benefits which he considers appropriate as a minimum for a basic hospital contract in his state. It should be an underlying principle for the establishment of any such benefits that the amounts are to be minimums, not maximums. In order to accommodate those states which have a substantial differential in hospital room and board costs between urban and rural areas within a state, the following language may be used in addition to the language in B(1) above: "except that $[insert amount] may be reduced to $[insert amount] outside the area." Other dollar amounts and percentage applicable to the various minimum benefits which follow are also bracketed to permit a commissioner to set the level of minimum benefits for his particular state.

(2) Miscellaneous hospital services for expenses incurred for the charges made by the hospital for services and supplies which are customarily rendered by the hospital and provided for use only during any one period of confinement in an amount not less than either [80%] of the charges incurred up to at least [$1,000] or [ten times] the daily hospital room and board benefits; and

(3) Hospital outpatient services consisting of (a) hospital services on the day surgery is performed, (b) hospital services rendered within seventy-two (72) hours after accidental injury, in an amount not less than [$50], and (c) X-ray and laboratory tests to the extent that benefits for such services would have been provided to an extent of less than [$100] if rendered to an in-patient of the hospital.

APPENDIX B

(4) Benefits provided under (1) and (2) of (B) above, may be provided subject to a combined deductible amount not in excess of [$100].

C. Basic Medical-Surgical Expense Coverage

"Basic Medical-Surgical Expense Coverage" is a policy of accident and sickness insurance which provides coverage for each person insured under the policy for the expenses incurred for the necessary services rendered by a physician for treatment of an injury or sickness for at least the following:

(1) Surgical services:

(a) In amounts not less than those provided on a fee schedule based on the relative values contained in the State of New York Certified Surgical Fee Schedule, or the 1964 California Relative Value Schedule or other acceptable relative value scale of surgical procedures, up to a maximum of at least [$500] for any one procedure; or

(b) Not less than [80%] of the reasonable charges.

(2) Anesthesia services, consisting of administration of necessary general anesthesia and related procedures in connection with covered surgical service rendered by a physician other than the physician (or his assistant) performing the surgical services:

(a) In an amount not less than [80%] of the reasonable charges; or

(b) [15%] of the surgical service benefit.

(3) In-hospital medical services, consisting of physician services rendered to a person who is a bed patient in a hospital for treatment of sickness or injury other than that for which surgical care is required, in an amount not less than [80%] of the reasonable charges; or [$5] per day for not less than twenty-one (21) days during one period of confinement.

D. Hospital Confinement Indemnity Coverage

"Hospital Confinement Indemnity coverage" is a policy of accident and sickness insurance which provides daily benefits for hospital confinement on an indemnity basis in an amount not less than [$20] per day and not less than thirty-one (31) days during any one period of confinement for each person insured under the policy.

E. Major Medical Expense Coverage

"Major medical expense coverage" is an accident and sickness insurance policy which provide hospital, medical and surgical expense coverage, to an aggregate maximum of not less than [$10,000]; copayment by the covered person not to exceed twenty-five percent (25%) of covered charges; a deductible stated on a per person, per family, per illness, per benefit period, or per year basis, or a combination of such bases not to exceed five percent (5%) of the aggregate maximum limit under the policy, unless the policy is written to complement underlying hospital and medical insurance in which case such deductible may be increased by the amount of the benefits provided by such underlying insurance, for each covered person for at least:

(1) Daily hospital room and board expenses, prior to application of the copayment percentage, for not less than [$50] daily (or in lieu thereof the average daily cost of the semiprivate room rate in the area where the insured resides) for a period of not less than thirty-one (31) days during continuous hospital confinement;

(2) Miscellaneous hospital services, prior to application of the copayment percentage, for an aggregate maximum of not less than [$4,500] or [15] times the daily room and board rate if specified in dollar amounts;

(3) Surgical services, prior to application of the copayment percentage to a maximum of not less than [$600] for the most severe operation with the amounts provided for other operations reasonably related to such maximum amount;

(4) Anesthesia services prior to application of the copayment percentage, for a maximum of not less than [15] percent of the covered surgical fees or, alternatively, if the surgical schedule is based on relative values, not less than the amount provided therein for anesthesia services at the same unit value as used for the surgical schedule;

(5) In-hospital medical services, prior to application of the co-payment percentage, as defined in Section 7C(3);

(6) Out-of-hospital care prior to application of the copayment percentage, consisting of physicians' services rendered on an ambulatory basis where coverage is not provided elsewhere in the policy for diagnosis and treatment of sickness or injury, and diagnostic x-ray, laboratory services, radiation therapy, and hemodialysis ordered by a physician; and

(7) Not fewer than three of the following additional benefits, prior to application of the copayment percentage, for an aggregate maximum of such covered charges of not less than [$1,000]:

    (a) In-hospital private duty graduate registered nurse services;

    (b) Convalescent nursing home care;

    (c) Diagnosis and treatment by a radiologist or physiotherapist;

(d) Rental of special medical equipment, as defined by the insurer in the policy;

(e) Artificial limbs or eyes, casts, splints, trusses or braces;

(f) Treatment for functional nervous disorders, and mental and emotional disorders; or

(g) Out-of-hospital prescription drugs and medications.

F. Disability Income Protection Coverage

"Disability income protection coverage" is a policy which provides for periodic payments, weekly or monthly, for a specified period during the continuance of disability resulting from either sickness or injury or a combination thereof which:

(1) Provides that periodic payments which are payable at ages after sixty-two (62) and reduced solely on the basis of age are at least fifty percent (50%) of amounts payable immediately prior to sixty-two.

(2) Contains an elimination period no greater than:

(a) Ninety (90) days in the case of a coverage providing a benefit of one (1) year or less;

(b) One hundred and eighty (180) days in the case of coverage providing a benefit of more than one year but not greater than two (2) years, or

(c) Three hundred sixty five (365) days in all other cases during the continuance of disability resulting from sickness or injury.

(3) Has a maximum period of time for which it is payable during disability of at least six (6) months except in the case of a policy covering disability arising out of pregnancy, childbirth or miscarriage in which case the period for such disability may be one (1) month. No reduction in benefits shall be put into effect because of an increase in Social Security or similar benefits during a benefit period. Section 7F does not apply to those policies providing business buy-out coverage.

G. Accident Only Coverage

"Accident-only coverage" is a policy of accident insurance which provides coverage, singly or in combination, for death, dismemberment, disability, or hospital and medical care caused by accident. Accidental death and double dismemberment amounts under such a policy shall be at least [$1,000] and a single dismemberment amount shall be at least [$500].

H. Specified Disease and Specified Accident Coverage

(1) "Specified disease coverage" pays benefits for the diagnosis and treatment of a specifically named disease or diseases. Any such policy must meet the following rules and one of the following sets of minimum standards for benefits; such insurance covering cancer--whether cancer only or in conjunction with other conditions(s) or disease(s)--must meet the standards of Subparagraph (c), (d), or (e); insurance covering specified disease(s) other than cancer must meet the standards of Subparagraph (b) or (e).

(a) General Rules

Except for cancer coverage provided on an expense-incurred basis, either as cancer-only coverage or in combination with one or more other specified diseases, the following rules shall apply to specified disease coverages in addition to all other rules imposed by this regulation; in cases of conflict between the following and other rules, the following ones shall govern:

(i) Policies covering a single specified disease or combination of specified diseases may not be sold or offered for sale other than as specified disease coverage under this section.

(ii) Any policy issued pursuant to this section which conditions payment upon pathological diagnosis of a covered disease, shall also provide that if such a pathological diagnosis is medically inappropriate, a clinical diagnosis will be accepted in lieu thereof.

(iii) Notwithstanding any other provision of this regulation, pecified disease policies shall provide benefits to any covered person not only for the specified disease(s) but also for any other conditions(s) or disease(s), directly caused or aggravated by the specified diseases(s) or the treatment of the specified disease(s).

(iv) Policies containing specified disease coverage shall be at least Guaranteed Renewable.

(v) No policy issued pursuant to this section shall contain a waiting or probationary period greater than thirty (30) days.

(vi) Any application for specified disease coverage shall contain a statement above the signature of the applicant that no person to be covered for specified disease is also covered by any Title XIX program (Medicaid, MediCal

APPENDIX B

    or any similar name). Such statement may be combined with any other statement for which the insurer may require the applicant's signature.

(vii) Payments may be conditioned upon a covered person's receiving medically necessary care, given in a medically appropriate location, under a medically accepted course of diagnosis or treatment.

(viii) Except for the uniform provision regarding other insurance with this insurer, benefits for specified disease coverage shall be paid regardless of other coverage available through individual health insurance.

Drafting Note: Specified disease coverage is recognized as supplemental coverage. Any specified disease coverage, therefore, must be payable in addition to and regardless of other individual coverage. The same general rule should apply so that group insurance cannot reduce its benefits because of the existence of an individual specified disease policy. Section 3F of the Group Coordination of Benefits Model Regulation states that the definition of a "plan" (for the purpose of COB) "shall not include individual or family insurance contracts..." It is recommended that states use this language to prevent benefit reductions that could otherwise occur because of the existence of an individual specified disease policy purchased by the insured.

(ix) After the effective date of the coverage (or applicable waiting period, it any) benefits shall begin with the first day of care or confinement if such care or confinement is for a covered disease even though the diagnosis is made at some later date. The retroactive application of such coverage may not be less than ninety (90) days prior to such diagnosis.

(b) The following minimum benefits standards apply to noncancer coverages:

(i) Coverage for each person insured under the policy for a specifically named disease (or diseases) with a deductible amount not in excess of [$250] and an overall aggregate benefit limit of no less than [$5,000] and a benefit period of not less than [two (2) years] for at least the following incurred expenses.

(A) Hospital room and board and any other hospital furnished medical services or supplies;

(B) Treatment by a legally qualified physician or surgeon;

(C) Private duty services of a registered nurse (R.N.);

(D) X-ray, radium and other therapy procedures used in diagnosis and treatment;

(E) Professional ambulance for local service to or from a local hospital;

(F) Blood transfusions, including expense incurred for blood donors;

(G) Drugs and medicines prescribed by a physician;

(H) The rental of an iron lung or similar mechanical apparatus;

(I) Brace, crutches and wheel chairs as are deemed necessary by the attending physician for the treatment of the disease;

(J) Emergency transportation if in the opinion of the attending physician it is necessary to transport the insured to another locality for treatment of the disease; and

(K) May include coverage of any other expenses necessarily incurred in the treatment of the disease.

(ii) Coverage for each person insured under the policy for a specifically named disease (or diseases) with no deductible amount, and an overall aggregate benefit limit of not less than [$25,000] payable at the rate of not less than [$50] a day while confined in a hospital and a benefit period of not less than 500 days.

(c) A policy which provides coverage for each person insured under the policy for cancer-only coverage or in combination with one or more other specified diseases on an expense incurred basis for services, supplies, care and treatment of cancer, in amounts not in excess of the usual and customary charges, with a deductible amount not in excess of [$250], and an overall aggregate benefit limit of not less than [$10,000] and a benefit period of not less than three (3) years for at least the following:

(i) Treatment by, or under the direction of, a legally qualified physician or surgeon;

(ii) X-ray, radium chemotherapy and other therapy procedures used in diagnosis and treatment;

APPENDIX B

(iii) Hospital room and board and any other hospital furnished medical services or supplies;

(iv) Blood transfusions, and the administration thereof, including expense incurred for blood donors;

(v) Drugs and medicines prescribed by a physician;

(vi) Professional ambulance for local service to or from a local hospital;

(vii) Private duty services of a registered nurse (R.N.) provided in a hospital;

(viii) May include coverage of any other expenses necessarily incurred in the treatment of the disease; provided however, that Items (i), (ii), (iv), (v) and (vii) plus at least the following shall also be included, but may be subject to copayment by the covered person not to exceed twenty percent (20%) of covered charges when rendered on an out-patient basis;

(ix) Braces, crutches and wheelchairs as are deemed necessary by the attending physician for the treatment of the disease;

(x) Emergency transportation if in the opinion of the attending physician in its necessary to transport the insured to another locality for treatment of the disease; and

(xi) Home health care that is necessary care and treatment provided at the covered person's residence by a home health care agency or by others under arrangements made with a home health care agency. The program of treatment must be prescribed in writing by the covered person's attending physician, who must approve the program prior to its start. The physician must certify that hospital confinement would be otherwise required. A "home health care agency" is (1) an agency approved under Title XVIII of the Social Security Act (Medicare), or (2) is licensed to provide home health care under applicable state law, or (3) meets all of the following requirements:

(A) It is primarily engaged in providing home health care services;

SUPPLEMENTAL HEALTH INSURANCE

  (B) Its policies are established by a group of professional personnel (including at least one physician and one registered nurse (R.N.);

  (C) Supervision of home health care services is provided by a physician or a registered nurse (R.N.);

  (D) It maintains clinical records on all patients; and

  (E) It has a full time administrator.

Drafting Note: State licensing laws vary concerning the scope of "home health care" or "home health agency services" and should be consulted. In addition, a few states have mandated benefits for home health care including the definition of required services.

  Home health includes, but is not limited to:

  (A) Part-time or intermittent skilled nursing services provided by a registered nurse (R.N.) or a licensed practical nurse (L.P.N.);

  (B) Part-time or intermittent home health aide services which provide supportive services in the home under the supervision of a registered nurse or a physical, speech or hearing occupational therapists;

  (C) Physical, occupational or speech and hearing therapy; and

  (D) Medical supplies, drugs and medicines prescribed by a physician and related pharmaceutical services, and laboratory services to the extent such charges or costs would have been covered under the policy if the insured person had remained in the hospital.

  (xii) Physical, speech, hearing and occupational therapy;

  (xiii) Special equipment including hospital bed, toilette, pulleys, wheelchairs, aspirator, chux, oxygen, surgical dressings, rubber shields, colostomy and eleostomy appliances;

  (xiv) Prosthetic devices including wigs and artificial breasts;

  (xv) Nursing home care for noncustodial services.

  (d) The following minimum benefits standards apply to cancer coverages written on a per diem indemnity basis. Such coverages must offer covered persons:

(i) A fixed-sum payment of at least [$100] for each day of hospital confinement for at least [365] days.

(ii) A fixed-sum payment equal to one half the hospital inpatient benefit for each day of hospital or nonhospital outpatient surgery, chemo- and radiation therapy, for at least 365 days of treatment.

Benefits tied to confinement in a skilled nursing home or to receipt of home health care are optional; if a policy offers these benefits, they must equal the following;

(iii) A fixed-sum payment equal to one-fourth the hospital in-patient benefit for each day of skilled nursing home confinement for at least 100 days.

(iv) A fixed-sum payment equal to one-fourth the hospital inpatient benefit for each day of home health care for at least 100 days.

(v) Benefit payments shall begin with the first day of care or confinement after the effective date of coverage if such care or confinement is for a covered disease even though the diagnosis of a covered disease is made at some later date (but not retroactive more than thirty (30) days from the date of diagnosis) if the initial care or confinement was for diagnosis or treatment of such covered disease.

(vi) Notwithstanding any other provision of this regulation, any restriction or limitation applied to the benefits in (d) (iii) and (d) (iv), whether by definition or otherwise, shall be no more restrictive than those under Medicare.

(e) The following minimum benefits standards apply to lump-sum indemnity coverage of any specified disease(s):

(i) Such coverages must pay indemnity benefits on behalf of covered persons of a specifically named disease or diseases. Such benefits are payable as a fixed, one-time payment made within thirty (30) days of submission to the insurer of proof of diagnosis of the specified disease(s). Dollar benefits shall be offered for sale only in even increments of $1,000.

SUPPLEMENTAL HEALTH INSURANCE

Drafting Note: Policies that offer extremely high dollar benefits may induce fraud and concealment on the part of applicants for coverage. Commissioners should be sensitive to this possibility in approving policies.

    (ii) Where coverage is advertised or otherwise represented to offer generic coverage of a disease or diseases, the same dollar amounts must be payable regardless of the particular subtype of the disease with one exception. In the case of clearly identifiable subtypes with significantly lower treatments costs, lesser amounts may be payable so long as the policy clearly differentiates that subtype and its benefits.

Drafting Note: The purpose of requiring equal coverage for all subtypes of a specified disease is to ensure that specified disease policies actually provide what people reasonable expect them to. In approving skin cancer or other exceptions, commissioners should consider whether a specified disease policy might mislead if it treats a subtype of a disease differently from the rest of the specified disease.

    (2) "Specified Accident coverage" is an accident insurance policy which provides coverage for a specifically identified kind of accident (or accidents) for each person insured under the policy for accidental death or accidental death and dismemberment, combined with a benefit amount not less than [$1,000] for accidental death, [$1,000] for double dismemberment [$500] for single dismemberment.

I. Limited Benefit Insurance Coverage

"Limited Benefit Health Insurance Coverage" is any policy or contract, other than a policy or contract covering only a specified disease or diseases, which provides benefits that are less than the minimum standards for benefits required under Section 7B, C, D, E, G, and H. A policy covering a single specified disease or combination of diseases shall meet the requirements of Section 7H and shall not be offered for sale as a "Limited Coverage." Such policies or contracts may be delivered or issued for delivery in this state only if the outline of coverage required by Section 8H of this regulation is completed and delivered as required by Section 8B of this regulation. This subsection does not apply to policies designed to provide coverage for long-term care or Medicare supplements, as defined in [cite provisions of Long-Term Care Act and Medicare Supplement Insurance Minimum Standards Act].

Section 8. **Required Disclosure Provisions**

    A. General Rules

        (1) Each individual policy of accident and sickness insurance or hospital, medical or dental service corporation subscriber contract shall include a renewal, continuation or nonrenewal provision. The language or

specification of such provision must be consistent with the type of contract to be issued. Such provision shall be appropriately captioned, shall appear on the first page of the policy, and shall clearly state the duration, where limited, of renewability and the duration of the term of coverage for which the policy is issued and for which it may be renewed.

(2) Except for riders or endorsements by which the insurer effectuates a request made in writing by the policyholder or exercises a specifically reserved right under the policy, all riders or endorsements added to a policy after date of issue or at reinstatement or renewal which reduce or eliminate benefits or coverage in the policy shall require signed acceptance by the policyholder. After date of policy issue, any rider or endorsement which increases benefits or coverage with a concomitant increase in premium during the policy term must be agreed to in writing signed by the insured, except if the increased benefits or coverage is required by law.

(3) Where a separate additional premium is charged for benefits provided in connection with riders or endorsements, such premium charge shall be set forth in the policy.

(4) A policy which provides for the payment of benefits based on standards described as "usual and customary," "reasonable and customary," or words of similar import shall include a definition of such terms and an explanation of such terms in its accompanying outline of coverage.

(5) If a policy contains any limitations with respect to preexisting conditions, such limitations must appear as a separate paragraph of the policy and be labeled as "Preexisting Condition Limitations."

(6) All accident-only policies shall contain ~~a prominent statement~~ on the first page of the policy or attached thereto in either contrasting color or in boldface type at least equal to the size of type used for policy captions, a prominent statement as follows:

"This is an accident-only policy and it does not pay benefits for loss from sickness."

(7) All policies, except single-premium nonrenewable policies and as otherwise provided in this paragraph, shall have a notice prominently printed on the first page of the policy or attached thereto stating in substance that the policyholder shall have the right to return the policy within ten (10) days of its delivery and to have the premium refunded if, after examination of the policy, the policyholder is not satisfied for any reason.

Drafting Note: This section should be included only if state has proper legislation.

(8) If age is to be used as a determining factor for reducing the maximum

SUPPLEMENTAL HEALTH INSURANCE

aggregate benefits made available in the policy as originally issued, such fact must be prominently set forth in the outline of coverage.

(9) If a policy contains a conversion privilege, it shall comply, in substance, with the following: The caption of the provision shall be "Conversion Privilege" or words of similar import. The provision shall indicate the persons eligible for conversion, the circumstances applicable to the conversion privilege, including any limitations on the conversion, and the person by whom the conversion privilege may be exercised. The provision shall specify the benefits to be provided on conversion or may state that the converted coverage will be as provided on a policy form then being used by the insurer for that purpose.

(10) Outlines of coverage delivered in connection with policies defined in this regulation as hospital confinement indemnity (Section 7D), Specified Disease (Section 7H), or Limited Benefit Health Insurance Coverages (Section 7I) to persons eligible for Medicare by reason of age shall contain, in addition to the requirements of subsections 8F and 8J, the following language which shall be printed on or attached to the first page of the outline of coverage:

This policy IS NOT A MEDICARE SUPPLEMENT policy. If you are eligible for Medicare, review the Medicare Supplement Buyer's Guide available from the company.

(11) Insurers, except direct response insurers, shall give any person applying for specified disease insurance a Buyer's Guide approved by the commissioner at the time of application and shall obtain all recipients' written acknowledgement of the guide's delivery. Direct response insurers shall provide the Buyer's Guide upon request but not later than the time the policy is delivered.

(12) All specified disease policies shall contain a prominent statement on the first page of the policy or attached thereto in either contrasting color or in boldface type at least equal to the size type used for policy captions, a prominent statement as follows: CAUTION: This is a limited policy. Read it carefully with the outline of coverage and the Buyer's Guide.

Drafting Note: The second sentence of this caption should only be required in those states where the commissioner exercises his discretionary authority and requires such guide.

B. Outline of Coverage Requirements for Individual Coverages

No individual accident and sickness insurance policy or nonprofit hospital, medical or dental service corporation subscriber contract subject to this regulation shall be delivered or issued for delivery in this state unless an appropriate outline of coverage, as prescribed in Section 8C through K is completed as to such policy or contract and the outline is either:

(1) Delivered with the policy; or

(2) Delivered to the applicant at the time application is made and acknowledgement of receipt or certification of delivery of such outline of coverage is provided to the insurer.

If an outline of coverage was delivered at the time of application and the policy or contract is issued on a basis which would require revision of the outline, a substitute outline of coverage properly describing the policy or contract must accompany the policy or contract when it is delivered and contain the following statement in no less than twelve (12) point type, immediately above the company name:

"NOTICE: Read this outline of coverage carefully. It is not identical to the outline of coverage provided upon application, and the coverage originally applied for has not been issued."

The appropriate outline of coverage for policies or contracts providing hospital coverage which only meets the standards of Section 7B shall be that statement contained in Section 8C. The appropriate outline of coverage for policies providing coverage which meets the standards of both Sections 7B and C shall be the statement contained in Section 8E. The appropriate outline of coverage for policies providing coverage which meets the standards of both Sections 7B and E or Section 7C and E or Section 7B, C, and E shall be the statement contained in Section 8G.

Appropriate changes in terminology may be made in the outline of coverage in the case of contracts of hospital, medical or dental service corporations. In any other case where the prescribed outline of coverage is inappropriate for the coverage provided by the policy or contract, an alternate outline of coverage shall be submitted to the commissioner for prior approval.

C. Basic Hospital Expense Coverage (Outline of Coverage)

An outline of coverage, in the form prescribed below, shall be issued in connection with policies meeting the standards of Section 7B of this regulation. The items included in the outline of coverage must appear in the sequence prescribed:

[COMPANY NAME]

BASIC HOSPITAL EXPENSE COVERAGE

OUTLINE OF COVERAGE

(1) Read Your Policy Carefully -- This outline of coverage provides a very brief description of the important features of your policy. This is not the

SUPPLEMENTAL HEALTH INSURANCE

insurance contract and only the actual policy provisions will control. The policy itself sets forth in detail the rights and obligations of both you and your insurance company. It is, therefore, important that you READ YOUR POLICY CAREFULLY!

(2) Basic Hospital Coverage -- Policies of this category are designed to provide, to persons insured, coverage for hospital expenses incurred as a result of a covered accident or sickness. Coverage is provided for daily hospital room and board, miscellaneous hospital services and hospital outpatient services, subject to any limitations, deductibles and copayment requirements set forth in the policy. Coverage is not provided for physicians or surgeons fees or unlimited hospital expenses.

(3) [A brief specific description of the benefits, including dollar amounts and number of days duration where applicable, contained in this policy, in the following order:

(a) Daily hospital room and board;

(b) Miscellaneous hospital services;

(c) Hospital out-patient services; and

(d) Other benefits, if any.]

Note: The above description of benefits shall be stated clearly and concisely, and shall include a description of any deductible or copayment provision applicable to the benefits described.

(4) [A description of any policy provisions which exclude, eliminate, restrict, reduce, limit, delay or in any other manner operate to qualify payment of the benefits described in (3) above.]

(5) [A description of policy provisions respecting renewability or continuation of coverage, including age restrictions or any reservation of right to change premiums.]

D. Basic Medical-Surgical Expense Coverage (Outline of Coverage)

An outline of coverage, in the form prescribed below, shall be issued in connection with policies meeting the standards of Section 7C of this regulation. The items included in the outline of coverage must appear in the sequence prescribed:

[COMPANY NAME]

BASIC MEDICAL-SURGICAL EXPENSE COVERAGE

OUTLINE OF COVERAGE

APPENDIX B

(1) Read Your Policy Carefully -- This outline of coverage provides a very brief description of the important features of your policy. This is not the insurance contract and only the actual policy provisions will control your policy. The policy itself sets forth in detail the rights and obligations of both you and your insurance company. It is, therefore, important that you READ YOUR POLICY CAREFULLY!

(2) Basic Medical-Surgical Expense Coverage--Policies of this category are designed to provide, to persons insured, coverage for medical-surgical expenses incurred as a result of a covered accident or sickness. Coverage is provided for surgical services, anesthesia services and in-hospital medical services, subject to any limitations, deductibles and copayment requirements set forth in the policy. Coverage is not provided for hospital expenses fees or unlimited medical-surgical expenses.

(3) [A brief specific description of the benefits, including dollar amounts and number of days duration where applicable, contained in this policy, in the following order:

(a) surgical services;

(b) anesthesia services;

(c) in-hospital medical services; and

(d) other benefits, if any]

Note: The above description of benefits shall be stated clearly and concisely, and shall include a description of any deductible or copayment provision applicable to the benefits described.

(4) [A description of any policy provisions which exclude, eliminate, restrict, reduce, limit, delay or in any other manner operate to qualify payment of the benefits described in (3) above.]

(5) [A description of policy provisions respecting renewability or continuation of coverage, including age restrictions or any reservation of right to change premiums.]

E. Basic Hospital and Medical-Surgical Expense Coverage (Outline of Coverage)

An outline of coverage, in the form prescribed below, shall be issued in connection with policies meeting the standards of Section 7B and C of this regulation. The items included in the outline of coverage must appear in the sequence prescribed.

[COMPANY NAME]

BASIC HOSPITAL AND MEDICAL-SURGICAL EXPENSE COVERAGE

OUTLINE OF COVERAGE

SUPPLEMENTAL HEALTH INSURANCE

(1) Read Your Policy Carefully -- This outline of coverage provides a very brief description of the important features of your policy. This is not the insurance contract and only the actual policy provisions will control. The policy itself sets forth in detail the rights and obligations of both you and your insurance company. It is, therefore important that your READ YOUR POLICY CAREFULLY!

(2) Basic Hospital and Medical-Surgical Expense Coverage -- Policies of this category are designed to provide, to persons insured, coverage for hospital and medical-surgical expenses incurred as a result of a covered accident or sickness. Coverage is provided for daily hospital room and board, miscellaneous hospital services, hospital out-patient services, surgical services, anesthesia services, and in-hospital medical services, subject to any limitations, deductibles and copayment requirements set forth in the policy. Coverage is not provided for unlimited hospital or medical surgical expenses.

(3) [A brief specific description of the benefits, including dollar amounts and number of days duration where applicable, contained in this policy, in the following order:

  (a) Daily hospital room and board;

  (b) Miscellaneous hospital services;

  (c) Hospital out-patient services;

  (d) Surgical services;

  (e) Anesthesia services;

  (f) In-hospital medical services; and

  (g) Other benefits, if any.]

Note: The above description of benefits shall be stated clearly and concisely, and shall include a description of any deductible or copayment provision applicable to the benefits described.

(4) [A description of any policy provisions which exclude, eliminate, restrict, reduce, limit, delay or in any other manner operate to qualify payment of the benefits described in (3) above.]

(5) [A description of policy provisions respecting renewability or continuation of coverage, including age restrictions or any reservation of right to change premiums.]

APPENDIX B

F. Hospital Confinement Indemnity Coverage (Outline of Coverage)

An outline of coverage, in the form prescribed below, shall be issued in connection with policies meeting the standards of Section 7D of this regulation. The items included in the outline of coverage must appear in the sequence prescribed:

[COMPANY NAME]

HOSPITAL CONFINEMENT INDEMNITY COVERAGE

OUTLINE OF COVERAGE

(1) Read Your Policy Carefully -- This outline of coverage provides a very brief description of the important feature of your policy. This is not the insurance contract and only the actual policy provisions will control. The policy itself sets forth in detail the rights and obligations of both you and your insurance company. It is, therefore, important that you READ YOUR POLICY CAREFULLY!

(2) Hospital Confinement Indemnity Coverage -- Policies of this category are designed to provide, to persons insured, coverage in the form of a fixed daily benefit during periods of hospitalization resulting from a covered accident or sickness, subject to any limitations set forth in the policy. Such policies do not provide any benefits other than the fixed daily indemnity for hospital confinement and any additional benefit described below.

(3) [A brief specific description of the benefits contained in this policy, in the following order:

(a) Daily benefit payable during hospital confinement; and

(b) Duration of benefit described in (a).]

Note: The above description of benefits shall be stated clearly and concisely.

(4) [A description of any policy provisions which exclude, eliminate, restrict, reduce, limit, delay or in any other manner operate to qualify payment of the benefit, described in (3) above.]

(5) [A description of policy provisions respecting renewability or continuation of coverage, including age restrictions or any reservation of right to change premiums.]

(6) [Any benefits provided in addition to the daily hospital benefit.]

G. Major Medical Expense Coverage (Outline of Coverage)

An outline of coverage, in the form prescribed below, shall be issued in connection with policies meeting the standards of Section 7E of this regulation.

The items included in the outline of coverage must appear in the sequence prescribed:

[COMPANY NAME]

MAJOR MEDICAL EXPENSE COVERAGE

OUTLINE OF COVERAGE

(1) Read Your Policy Carefully -- This outline of coverage provides a very brief description of the important features of your policy. This is not the insurance contract and only the actual policy provisions will control. The policy itself sets forth in detail the rights and obligations of both you and your insurance company. It is, therefore, important that you READ YOUR POLICY CAREFULLY!

(2) Major Medical Expense Coverage -- Policies of this category are designed to provide, to persons insured, coverage for major hospital, medical, and surgical expenses incurred as a result of a covered accident or sickness. Coverage is provided for daily hospital room and board, miscellaneous hospital services, surgical services, anesthesia services, in-hospital medical services, and out-of-hospital care, subject to any deductibles, copayment provisions, or other limitations which may be set forth in the policy. Basic hospital or basic medical insurance coverage is not provided.

(3) [A brief specific description of the benefits, including dollar amounts, contained in this policy, in the following order:

    (a) Daily hospital room and board;

    (b) Miscellaneous hospital services,

    (c) Surgical services;

    (d) Anesthesia services;

    (e) In-hospital medical services,

    (f) Out-of-hospital care;

    (g) Maximum dollar amount for covered charges; and

    (h) Other benefits, if any]

Note: The above description of benefits shall be stated clearly and concisely, and shall include a description of any deductible or copayment provision applicable to the benefits described.

(4) [A description of any policy provision which exclude, eliminate, restrict,

APPENDIX B

    reduce, limit, delay or in any other manner operate to qualify payment of the benefits described in (3) above.]

  (5) [A description of policy provisions respecting renewability or continuation of coverage, including age restrictions or any reservation of right to change premiums.]

H. Disability Income Protection Coverage (Outline of Coverage)

An outline of coverage, in the form prescribed below, shall be issued in connection with policies meeting the standards of Section 7F of this regulation. The items included in the outline of coverage must appear in the sequence prescribed:

[COMPANY NAME]

DISABILITY INCOME PROTECTION COVERAGE

OUTLINE OF COVERAGE

(1) Read Your Policy Carefully -- This outline of coverage provides a very brief description of the important features of your policy. This is not the insurance contract and only the actual policy provisions will control. The policy itself sets forth in detail the rights and obligations of both you and your insurance company. It is, therefore, important that you READ YOUR POLICY CAREFULLY!

(2) Disability Income protection Coverage -- Policies of this category are designed to provide, to persons insured, coverage for disabilities resulting from a covered accident or sickness, subject to any limitations set forth in the policy. Coverage is not provided for basic hospital, basic medical-surgical, or major medical expenses.

(3) [A brief specific description of the benefits contained in this policy:]

Note: The above description of benefits shall be stated clearly and concisely.

(4) [A description of any policy provisions which exclude, eliminate, restrict, reduce, limit, delay or in any other manner operate to qualify payment of the benefits described in (3) above.]

(5) [A description of policy provisions respecting renewability or continuation of coverage, including age restrictions or any reservation of right to change premiums.]

SUPPLEMENTAL HEALTH INSURANCE

I. Accident-Only Coverage (Outline of Coverage)

An outline of coverage in the form prescribed below, shall be issued in connection with policies meeting the standards of Section 7G of this regulation. The items included in the outline of coverage must appear in the sequence prescribed:

[COMPANY NAME]

ACCIDENT-ONLY COVERAGE

OUTLINE OF COVERAGE

(1) Read Your Policy Carefully -- This outline of coverage provides a very brief description of the important features of your policy. This is not the insurance contract and only the actual policy provisions will control. The policy itself sets forth in detail the rights and obligations of both you and your insurance company. It is, therefore, important that you READ YOUR POLICY CAREFULLY!

(2) Accident-Only coverage -- Policies of this category are designed to provide, to persons insured, coverage for certain losses resulting from a covered accident ONLY, subject to any limitations contained in the policy. Coverage is not provided for basic hospital, basic medical-surgical, or major medical expenses.

(3) [A brief specific description of the benefits contained in this policy.]

Note: The above description of benefits shall be stated clearly and concisely, and shall include a description of any deductible or copayment provision applicable to the benefits described. Proper disclosure of benefits which vary according to accidental cause shall be made in accordance with Section 7A(13) of this regulation.

(4) [A description of any policy provisions which exclude, eliminate, restrict, reduce, limit, delay or in any other manner operate to qualify payment of the benefits described in (3) above.]

(5) [A description of policy provisions respecting renewability or continuation of coverage, including age restrictions or any reservations of right to change premiums.]

J. Specified Disease or Specified Accident Coverage (Outline of Coverage)

An outline of coverage in the form prescribed below, shall be issued in connection with policies meeting the standards of Section 7H of this regulation. The coverage shall be identified by the appropriate bracketed title. The items included in the outline of coverage must appear in the sequence prescribed:

APPENDIX B

[COMPANY NAME]

[SPECIFIED DISEASE] [SPECIFIED ACCIDENT] COVERAGE

OUTLINE OF COVERAGE

(1) This policy is designed only as a supplement to a comprehensive health insurance policy and should not be purchased unless you have this underlying coverage. It should not be purchased by persons covered under Medicaid. Read the Buyer's Guide's discussion of the possible limits on benefits in this type of policy.

(2) Read Your Policy Carefully -- This outline of coverage provides a very brief description of the important features of your policy. This is not the insurance contract and only the actual policy provisions will control. The policy itself sets forth in detail the rights and obligations of both you and your insurance company. It is, therefore, important that you READ YOUR POLICY CAREFULLY!

(3) [Specified Disease] [Specified Accident] Coverage -- Policies of this category are designed to provide, to persons insured, restricted coverage paying benefits ONLY when certain losses occur as a result of [specified diseases] or [specified accidents]. Coverage is not provided for basic hospital, basic medical-surgical, or major medical expenses.

(4) [A brief specific description of the benefits, including dollar amounts, contained in this policy.]

Note: The above description of benefits shall be stated clearly and concisely, and shall include a description of any deductible or copayment provisions applicable to the benefits described. Proper disclosure of benefits which vary according to accidental cause shall be made in accordance with Section 7A(13) of this regulation.

K. Limited Benefit Health Coverage (Outline of Coverage)

An outline of coverage, in the form prescribed below, shall be issued in connection with policies which do not meet the minimum standards of Section 7B, C, D, E, F, G and H of this regulation. The items included in the outline of coverage must appear in the sequence prescribed:

[COMPANY NAME]

LIMITED BENEFIT HEALTH COVERAGE

OUTLINE OF COVERAGE

(1) Read Your Policy Carefully -- The outline of coverage provides a very brief description of the important features of your policy. This is not the

SUPPLEMENTAL HEALTH INSURANCE

insurance contract and only the actual policy provisions will control. The policy itself sets forth in detail the rights and obligations of both you and your insurance company. It is, therefore important that you READ YOUR POLICY CAREFULLY!

(2) Limited Benefit Health Coverage -- Policies of this category are designed to provide, to persons insured, limited or supplemental coverage.

(3) [A brief specific description of the benefits, including dollar amounts, contained in this policy.]

Note: The above description of benefits shall be stated clearly and concisely, and shall include a description of any deductible or copayment provisions applicable to the benefits described. Proper disclosure of benefits which vary according to accidental cause shall be made in accordance with Section 7A(13) of this regulation.

(4) [A description of any policy provisions which exclude, eliminate, restrict, reduce, limit, delay or in any other manner operate to qualify payment of the benefits described in (3) above.]

(5) [A description of policy provisions respecting renewability or continuation of coverage, including age restrictions or any reservations of right to change premiums.]

Section 9. **Requirements for Replacement**

A. Application forms shall include a question designed to elicit information as to whether the insurance to be issued is intended to replace any other accident and sickness insurance presently in force. A supplementary application or other form to be signed by the applicant containing such a questions may be used.

B. Upon determining that a sale will involve replacement, an insurer, other than a direct response insurer, or its agent shall furnish the applicant, prior to issuance or delivery of the policy, the notice described in C below. One (1) copy of such notice shall be retained by the insurer. A direct response insurer shall deliver to the applicant upon issuance of the policy, the notice described in D below. In no event, however, will such a notice be required in the solicitation of the following types of policies; accident-only and single-premium nonrenewable policies.

C. The notice required by B above for an insurer, other than a direct response insurer, shall provide, in substantially the following form:

NOTICE TO APPLICANT REGARDING REPLACEMENT

OF ACCIDENT AND SICKNESS INSURANCE

According to [your application] [information you have furnished], you intend to lapse or otherwise terminate existing accident and sickness insurance and replace it with a policy to be issued by [insert company name] Insurance Company. For your own information and protection, you should be aware of and seriously consider certain factors which may affect the insurance protection available to you under the new policy.

    (1)   Health conditions which you may presently have, (preexisting conditions) may not be immediately or fully covered under the new policy. This could result in denial or delay of a claim for benefits present under the new policy, whereas a similar claim might have been payable under your present policy.

Drafting Note: This subsection may be modified if preexisting conditions are covered under the new policy.

    (2)   You may wish to secure the advice of your present insurer or its agent regarding the proposed replacement of your present policy. This is not only your right, but it is also in your best interests to make sure you understand all the relevant factors involved in replacing your present coverage.

    (3)   If, after due consideration, you still wish to terminate your present policy and replace it with new coverage, be certain to truthfully and completely answer all questions on the application concern your medical/health history. Failure to include all material medical information on an application may provide a basis for the company to deny any future claims and to refund your premium as though your policy had never been in force. After the application has been completed and before you sign it, reread it carefully to be certain that all information has been properly recorded.

The above "Notice to Applicant" was delivered to me on:

_____
(Date)

_____
(Applicant's Signature)

    D.   The notice required by B above for a direct response insurer shall be as follows:

NOTICE TO APPLICANT REGARDING REPLACEMENT

OF ACCIDENT AND SICKNESS INSURANCE

According to [your application] [information you have furnished] you intend to lapse or otherwise terminate existing accident and sickness insurance and replace it with the policy delivered herewith issued by [insert company name] Insurance Company. Your new policy provides ten days within which you may decide without cost whether you desire to keep the policy. For your own information and protection you should be aware of and seriously consider certain factors which may affect the insurance protection available to you under the new policy.

(1) Health conditions which you may presently have, (preexisting conditions) may not be immediately or fully covered under the new policy. This could result in denial or delay of a claim for benefits under the new policy, whereas a similar claim might have been payable under your present policy.

(2) You may wish to secure the advice of your present insurer or its agent regarding the proposed replacement of your present policy. This is not only your right, but it is also in your best interests to make sure you understand all the relevant factors involved in replacing your present coverage.

(3) [To be included only if the application is attached to the policy]. If, after due consideration, you still wish to terminate your present policy and replace it with new coverage, read the copy of the application attached to your new policy and be sure that all questions are answered fully and correctly. Omissions or misstatements in the application could cause an otherwise valid claim to be denied. Carefully check the application and write to [insert company name and address] within ten days if any information is not correct and complete, or if any past medical history has been left out of the application.

[COMPANY NAME]

Section 10.   Separability

If any provision of this regulation or the application thereof to any person or circumstance is for any reason held to be invalid, the remainder of the regulation and the application of such provision to other persons or circumstances shall not be affected thereby.

Legislative History (all references are to the Proceedings of the NAIC).

1975 Proc. I 2, 6, 573, 575, 590-605 (adopted).
1977 Proc. I 26, 28, 54-77, 317, 325 (amended).
1979 Proc. II 31, 34, 327, 333, 339-344 (amended regarding Medicare supplement insurance).
1980 Proc. II 22, 26, 588, 591, 594, 622, 634-636 (amended).
1989 Proc. II 13, 23-24, 467-468, 518-519, 548-570 (amended to remove reference to Medicare supplement insurance).

Appendix C

MEDICARE SUPPLEMENT INSURANCE MINIMUM STANDARDS MODEL ACT

(Model Regulation Service—April 1995)

From the NAIC *Model Laws, Regulations and Guidelines.* Reprinted with permission of the National Association of Insurance Commissioners.

Table of Contents

Section 1. Definitions
Section 2. Applicability and Scope
Section 3. Standards for Policy Provisions and Authority to Promulgate Regulations
Section 4. Loss Ratio Standards
Section 5. Disclosure Standards
Section 6. Notice of Free Examination
Section 7. Filing Requirements for Advertising
Section 8. Administrative Procedures
Section 9. Penalties
Section 10. Separability
Section 11. Effective Date

Section 1. Definitions

 A. "Applicant" means:

  (1) In the case of an individual Medicare supplement policy, the person who seeks to contract for insurance benefits, and

  (2) In the case of a group Medicare supplement policy, the proposed certificateholder.

 B. "Certificate" means, for the purposes of this Act, any certificate delivered or issued for delivery in this state under a group Medicare supplement policy.

 C. "Certificate form" means the form on which the certificate is delivered or issued for delivery by the issuer.

 D. "Issuer" includes insurance companies, fraternal benefit societies, health care service plans, health maintenance organizations, and any other entity delivering or issuing for delivery in this state Medicare supplement policies or certificates.

Drafting Note: It is intended that nonprofit hospital and medical service associations be subject to this model act. In those states where such associations are prohibited from issuing subscriber contracts that include all of the benefits required by Section 3 of this Act, they shall include so much of those benefits as are permitted and they shall be issued in conjunction with another contract including at least the remainder of the minimum benefits required. In such event, the combination of contracts will be considered to have been issued in compliance with Section 3 of this Act.

 E. "Medicare" means the "Health Insurance for the Aged Act," Title XVIII of the Social Security Amendments of 1965, as then constituted or later amended.

 F. "Medicare supplement policy" means a group or individual policy of [accident and sickness] insurance or a subscriber contract [of hospital and medical service

SUPPLEMENTAL HEALTH INSURANCE

associations or health maintenance organizations], other than a policy issued pursuant to a contract under Section 1876 of the federal Social Security Act (42 U.S.C. Section 1395 et. seq.), or an issued policy under a demonstration project specified in 42 U.S.C. § 1395ss(g)(1), which is advertised, marketed or designed primarily as a supplement to reimbursements under Medicare for the hospital, medical or surgical expenses of persons eligible for Medicare.

Drafting Note: OBRA 1990 contained an exception from this definition for policies issued pursuant to an agreement under Section 1833 (42 U.S.C. 1395l) of the federal Social Security Act. The Social Security Act Amendments of 1994 eliminated the exemption for Section 1833 plans effective December 31, 1995. These plans, commonly know as health care prepayment plans (HCPPs), arrange for certain Part B services on a pre-paid basis. The federal law continues to authorize HCPP agreements. However, since they are now included in the federal definition of a Medicare supplement policy, HCPPs are subject to the requirements of this model, unless they are exempt under Section 2B. In states authorized for the Medicare Select program, these plans may be able to comply with Medicare supplement requirements.

    G.   "Policy form" means the form on which the policy is delivered or issued for delivery by the issuer.

Section 2. Applicability and Scope

    A.   Except as otherwise specifically provided this Act shall apply to:

        (1)   All Medicare supplement policies delivered or issued for delivery in this state on or after the effective date of this Act, and

        (2)   All certificates issued under group Medicare supplement policies, which certificates have been delivered or issued for delivery in this state.

    B.   This Act shall not apply to a policy of one or more employers or labor organizations, or of the trustees of a fund established by one or more employers or labor organizations, or combination thereof, for employees or former employees or a combination thereof, or for members or former members, or a combination thereof, of the labor organizations.

    C.   <u>Except as otherwise specifically provided in section 5D,</u> the provisions of this Act are not intended to prohibit or apply to insurance policies or health care benefit plans, including group conversion policies, provided to Medicare eligible persons when the policies are not marketed or held to be Medicare supplement policies or benefit plans.

Section 3. Standards for Policy Provisions and Authority to Promulgate Regulations

    A.   No Medicare supplement policy or certificate in force in the state shall contain benefits that duplicate benefits provided by Medicare.

    B.   Notwithstanding any other provision of law of this state, a Medicare supplement policy or certificate shall not exclude or limit benefits for loss incurred more than six (6) months from the effective date of coverage because it involved a preexisting condition. The policy or certificate shall not define a preexisting condition more restrictively than a condition for which medical advice was given or treatment was recommended by or received from a physician within six (6) months before the effective date of coverage.

    C.   The commissioner shall adopt reasonable regulations to establish specific standards for policy provisions of Medicare supplement policies and certificates. The standards shall be in addition to and in accordance with applicable laws of this state, including Sections [insert the applicable statutory reference, if any, to the NAIC Uniform Accident and Sickness Policy Provision Law]. No requirement of the Insurance Code relating to minimum required policy benefits, other than the minimum standards contained in this Act, shall apply to Medicare supplement policies and certificates. The standards may cover, but not be limited to:

Editor's Note: Wherever the term "commissioner" appears, the title of the chief insurance regulatory official of the state should be inserted.

    (1)   Terms of renewability;

    (2)   Initial and subsequent conditions of eligibility;

    (3)   Nonduplication of coverage;

    (4)   Probationary periods;

    (5)   Benefit limitations, exceptions and reductions;

    (6)   Elimination periods;

    (7)   Requirements for replacement;

    (8)   Recurrent conditions; and

    (9)   Definitions of terms.

D.   The commissioner shall adopt reasonable regulations to establish minimum standards for benefits, claims payment, marketing practices and compensation arrangements and reporting practices, for Medicare supplement policies and certificates.

E.   The commissioner may adopt from time to time reasonable regulations necessary to conform Medicare supplement policies and certificates to the requirements of federal law and regulations promulgated thereunder, including but not limited to:

    (1)   Requiring refunds or credits if the policies or certificates do not meet loss ratio requirements;

    (2)   Establishing a uniform methodology for calculating and reporting loss ratios;

    (3)   Assuring public access to policies, premiums and loss ratio information of issuers of Medicare supplement insurance;

    (4)   Establishing a process for approving or disapproving policy forms and certificate forms and proposed premium increases;

    (5)   Establishing a policy for holding public hearings prior to approval of premium increases; and

    (6)   Establishing standards for Medicare Select policies and certificates.

F.   The commissioner may adopt reasonable regulations that specify prohibited policy provisions not otherwise specifically authorized by statute which, in the opinion of the commissioner, are unjust, unfair or unfairly discriminatory to any person insured or proposed to be insured under a Medicare supplement policy or certificate.

Drafting Note: Each state should examine its statutory authority to promulgate regulations and revise this section accordingly so that sufficient rulemaking authority is present and that unnecessary duplication of unfair practice provisions does not occur.

Section 4. Loss Ratio Standards

Medicare supplement policies shall return to policyholders benefits which are reasonable in relation to the premium charged. The commissioner shall issue reasonable regulations to establish minimum standards for loss ratios of Medicare supplement policies on the basis of incurred claims experience, or incurred health care expenses where coverage is provided by a health maintenance organization on a service rather than reimbursement basis, and earned premiums in accordance with accepted actuarial principles and practices.

Section 5. Disclosure Standards

A. In order to provide for full and fair disclosure in the sale of Medicare supplement policies, no Medicare supplement policy or certificate shall be delivered in this state unless an outline of coverage is delivered to the applicant at the time application is made.

B. The commissioner shall prescribe the format and content of the outline of coverage required by Subsection A. For purposes of this section, "format" means style, arrangements and overall appearance, including such items as the size, color and prominence of type and arrangement of text and captions. The outline of coverage shall include:

(1) A description of the principal benefits and coverage provided in the policy;

(2) A statement of the renewal provisions, including any reservation by the issuer of a right to change premiums; and disclosure of the existence of any automatic renewal premium increases based on the policyholder's age.

(3) A statement that the outline of coverage is a summary of the policy issued or applied for and that the policy should be consulted to determine governing contractual provisions.

C. The commissioner may prescribe by regulation a standard form and the contents of an informational brochure for persons eligible for Medicare, which is intended to improve the buyer's ability to select the most appropriate coverage and improve the buyer's understanding of Medicare. Except in the case of direct response insurance policies, the commissioner may require by regulation that the informational brochure be provided to any prospective insureds eligible for Medicare concurrently with delivery of the outline of coverage. With respect to direct response insurance policies, the commissioner may require by regulation that the prescribed brochure be provided upon request to any prospective insureds eligible for Medicare, but in no event later than the time of policy delivery.

D. The commissioner may adopt regulations for captions or notice requirements, determined to be in the public interest and designed to inform prospective insureds that particular insurance coverages are not Medicare supplement coverages, for all accident and sickness insurance policies sold to persons eligible for Medicare, other than:

(1) Medicare supplement policies; or

(2) Disability income policies.

E. The commissioner may adopt reasonable regulations to govern the full and fair disclosure of the information in connection with the replacement of accident and sickness policies, subscriber contracts or certificates by persons eligible for Medicare.

Section 6. Notice of Free Examination

Medicare supplement policies and certificates shall have a notice prominently printed on the first page of the policy or certificate or attached thereto stating in substance that the applicant shall have the right to return the policy or certificate within thirty (30) days of its delivery and to have the premium refunded if, after examination of the policy or certificate, the applicant is not satisfied for any reason. A refund made pursuant to this section shall be paid directly to the applicant by the issuer in a timely manner.

Section 7. Filing Requirements for Advertising

Every issuer of Medicare supplement insurance policies or certificates in this state shall provide a copy of any Medicare supplement advertisement intended for use in this state whether through written, radio or television medium to the Commissioner of Insurance of this state for review or approval by the commissioner to the extent it may be required under state law.

Drafting Note: States should examine their existing laws regarding the filing of advertisements to determine the extent to which review or approval is required.

Section 8. Administrative Procedures

Regulations adopted pursuant to this Act shall be subject to the provisions of [cite section of state insurance code relating to the adoption and promulgation of rules and regulations or cite the state's administrative procedures act, if applicable].

Section 9. Penalties

In addition to any other applicable penalties for violations of the Insurance Code, the commissioner may require issuers violating any provision of this Act or regulations promulgated pursuant to this Act to cease marketing any Medicare supplement policy or certificate in this state which is related directly or indirectly to a violation or may require the issuer to take actions necessary to comply with the provisions of this Act, or both.

Section 10. Separability

If any provision of this Act or the application of it to any person or circumstances is for any reason held to be invalid, the remainder of the Act and the application of the provision to other persons or circumstances shall not be affected.

Section 11. Effective Date

The Act shall be effective on [insert date].

Legislative History (all references are to the Proceedings of the NAIC).

1980 Proc. II 22, 26, 588, 591, 593, 603-605 (adopted).
1981 Proc. I 47, 51, 420, 424, 446, 453-456 (amended and reprinted).
1988 Proc. I 9, 20-21, 629-630, 652-654, 665-668 (amended and reprinted).
1988 Proc. II 5, 13, 568, 601, 604, 624-626 (amended and reprinted).
1989 Proc. I 14, 813-814, 836.1-836.4 (amended at special plenary session September 1988).
1990 Proc. I 6, 27-28, 477, 574-575, 577-580 (amended and reprinted).
1992 Proc. I 12, 12-16, 1085 (amended at special plenary in July 1991).
1995 Proc. 1st Quarter 7, 12, 501, 575, 586, 588-591 (amended and reprinted).

Appendix D

RULES GOVERNING ADVERTISEMENTS OF ACCIDENT AND SICKNESS INSURANCE WITH INTERPRETIVE GUIDELINES

(Model Regulation Service—July 1989)

From the NAIC *Model Laws, Regulations and Guidelines*. Reprinted with permission of the National Association of Insurance Commissioners.

Table of Contents

Preamble
Section 1.   Purpose
Section 2.   Applicability
Section 3.   Definitions
Section 4.   Method of Disclosure of Required Information
Section 5.   Form and Content of Advertisements
Section 6.   Advertisement of Benefits Payable, Losses Covered by Premiums Payable
Section 7.   Necessity for Disclosing Policy Provisions Relating to Renewability, Cancellability and Termination
Section 8.   Testimonials or Endorsements by Third Parties
Section 9.   Use of Statistics
Section 10. Identification of Plan or Number of Policies
Section 11. Disparaging Comparisons and Statements
Section 12. Jurisdictional Licensing and Status of Insurer
Section 13. Identity of Insurer
Section 14. Group or Quasi-Group Implications
Section 15. Introductory, Initial or Special Offers
Section 16. Statements About an Insurer
Section 17. Enforcement Procedures
Section 18. Severability Provision
Section 19. Filing for Prior Review
Appendix   Interpretive Guidelines

Preamble

The proper expansion of accident and sickness coverage is in the public interest. Appropriate advertising can broaden the distribution of insurance and coverage under health maintenance organizations and other prepaid plans among various segments of the public. These rules, while referencing insurance, are intended to apply to the advertisement of accident and sickness benefits whether provided on an indemnity, reimbursement, service or prepaid basis. Advertising can increase public awareness of new and beneficial forms of coverage and thereby encourage product competition. Advertising can also provide the insurance-buying public with the means by which it can compare the advantages of competing forms of coverage.

Insurance advertising has become increasingly important in the years since the 1956 Rules Governing Advertising of Accident and Sickness Insurance were developed. The increasing availability of coverage under group insurance plans and the advent of governmental benefit programs have complicated the decisions the insurance-buying public must make to avoid duplication of benefits and gaps in coverage. The consequent need for detailed information about insurance products is reflected in the requirements for disclosure established by the 1972 Rules (as amended in 1977) Governing Advertisements of Accident and Sickness Insurance. This need for detailed disclosure is especially critical in helping to assure that the insurance-buying public receives full and truthful advertising for accident and sickness insurance. In 1987 the NAIC adopted the Model Rules Governing Advertisements of Medicare Supplement Insurance With Interpretive Guidelines to separately address Medicare supplement insurance advertising. The NAIC has now determined that while the 1972 Rules (as amended in 1977) Governing Advertisements of Accident and Sickness Insurance did address accident and sickness insurance, these new Rules and Interpretive Guidelines revise the previous 1972 Rules and Interpretive Guidelines with respect to accident and sickness insurance advertising and eliminate duplicative or inconsistent regulation of Medicare supplement insurance advertising.

Although modern insurance advertising patterns much of its design after advertising for other goods and services, the uniqueness of insurance as a product must always be kept in mind in developing advertising of accident and sickness insurance. By the time an insured discovers that a particular insurance product is unsuitable for his needs, it may be too late for him to return to the marketplace to find a more satisfactory product.

Hence, the insurance-buying public should be afforded a means by which it can determine, in advance of purchase, the desirability of the competing insurance products proposed to be sold. This can be accomplished by advertising which accurately describes the advantages and disadvantages of the insurance product without either exaggerating the benefits or minimizing the limitations. Properly designed advertising can provide such description and disclosure without sacrificing the sales appeal which is essential to its usefulness to the insurance-buying public and the insurance business. The purpose of the new Rules Governing Advertisements of Accident and Sickness Insurance is to establish minimum criteria to assure proper and accurate description and disclosure.

Section 1. Purpose

The purpose of these rules is to protect prospective purchasers with respect to the advertisement of accident and sickness insurance in the same manner as the rules governing advertisements of Medicare supplement insurance. The rules assure the clear and truthful disclosure of the benefits, limitations and exclusions of policies sold as accident and sickness insurance. This is intended to be accomplished by the establishment of guidelines and permissible and impermissible standards of conduct in the advertising of accident and sickness insurance in a manner which prevents unfair, deceptive and misleading advertising and is conducive to accurate presentation and description to the insurance-buying public through the advertising media and material used by insurance agents and companies.

Section 2. Applicability

A. These rules shall apply to any accident and sickness (except Medicare supplement insurance) "advertisement," as that term is defined herein unless otherwise specified in these rules, which the insurer knows or reasonably should know is intended for presentation, distribution or dissemination in this State when such presentation, distribution or dissemination is made either directly or indirectly by or on behalf of an insurer, agent, broker, producer or solicitor, as those terms are defined in the Insurance Code of this State.

B. Every insurer shall establish and at all times maintain a system of control over the content, form and method of dissemination of all advertisements of its policies. All such advertisements, regardless of by whom written, created, designed or presented, shall be the responsibility of the insurer whose policies are so advertised.

C. Advertising materials which are reproduced in quantity shall be identified by form numbers or other identifying means. Such identification shall be sufficient to distinguish an advertisement from any other advertising materials, policies, applications or other materials used by the insurer.

Section 3. Definitions

A. (1) An advertisement for the purpose of these rules shall include:

(a) Printed and published material, audio visual material, and descriptive literature of an insurer used in direct mail, newspapers, magazines, radio scripts, TV scripts, billboards and similar displays; and

(b) Descriptive literature and sales aids of all kinds issued by an insurer, agent, producer, broker or solicitor for presentation to members of the insurance-buying public, including but not limited to circulars, leaflets, booklets, depictions, illustrations, form letters and lead-generating devices of all kinds as herein defined; and

(c) Prepared sales talks, presentations and material for use by agents, brokers, producers and solicitors whether prepared by the insurer or the agent, broker, producer or solicitor.

(2) The definition of "advertisement" includes advertising material included with a policy when the policy is delivered and material used in the solicitation of renewals and reinstatements.

(3) The definition of "advertisement" does not include:

(a) Material to be used solely for the training and education of an insurer's employees, agents or brokers;

(b) Material used in-house by insurers;

(c) Communications within an insurer's own organization not intended for dissemination to the public;

(d) Individual communications of a personal nature with current policyholders other than material urging such policyholders to increase or expand coverages;

(e) Correspondence between a prospective group or blanket policyholder and an insurer in the course of negotiating a group or blanket contract;

(f) Court-approved material ordered by a court to be disseminated to policyholders; or

(g) A general announcement from a group or blanket policyholder to eligible individuals on an employment or membership list that a contract or program has been written or arranged; provided, the announcement clearly indicates that it is preliminary to the issuance of a booklet.

B. "Accident and Sickness Insurance Policy" for the purpose of these rules shall include any policy, plan, certificate, contract, agreement, statement of coverage, rider or endorsement which provides accident or sickness benefits or medical, surgical or hospital expense benefits, whether on an indemnity, reimbursement, service or prepaid basis, except when issued in connection with another kind of insurance other than life and except disability, waiver of premium and double indemnity benefits included in life insurance and annuity contracts. Accident and sickness insurance policy shall not include any Medicare supplement insurance policy.

C. "Certificate" means for the purpose of these rules, any certificate issued under a group accident and sickness insurance policy, which certificate has been delivered or issued for delivery in this State.

D. "Insurer" for the purpose of these rules shall include any individual, corporation, association, partnership, reciprocal exchange, inter-insurer, Lloyds, fraternal benefit society, health maintenance organization, hospital service corporation, medical service corporation, prepaid health plan and any other legal entity which is defined as an "insurer" in the Insurance Code of this State and is engaged in the advertisement of itself, or an accident and sickness insurance policy.

E. "Exception" for the purpose of these rules shall mean any provision in a policy whereby coverage for a specified hazard is entirely eliminated; it is a statement of a risk not assumed under the policy.

F. "Reduction" for the purpose of these rules shall mean any provision which reduces the amount of the benefit; a risk of loss is assumed but payment upon the occurrence of such loss is limited to some amount or period less than would be otherwise payable and such reduction has not been used.

G. "Limitation" for the purpose of these rules shall mean any provision which restricts coverage under the policy other than an exception or a reduction.

H. "Institutional Advertisement" for the purpose of these rules shall mean an advertisement having as its sole purpose the promotion of the reader's, viewer's or listener's interest in the concept of accident and sickness insurance, or the promotion of the insurer as a seller of accident and sickness insurance.

I. "Invitation to Inquire" for the purpose of these rules shall mean an advertisement having as its objective the creation of a desire to inquire further about accident and sickness insurance and which is limited to a brief description of coverage, and which shall contain a provision in the following or substantially similar form:

> "This policy has [exclusions] [limitations] [reduction of benefits] [terms under which the policy may be continued in force or discontinued]. For costs and complete details of the coverage, call [or write] your insurance agent or the company [whichever is applicable]."

J. "Invitation to Contract" for the purpose of these rules shall mean an advertisement which is neither an invitation to inquire nor an institutional advertisement.

K. "Person" for the purpose of these rules shall mean any natural person, association, organization, partnership, trust, group, discretionary group, corporation or any other entity.

L. "Lead-Generating Device", for the purpose of these rules, shall mean any communication directed to the public which, regardless of form, content or stated purpose, is intended to result in the compilation or qualification of a list containing names and other personal information to be used to solicit residents of this State for the purchase of accident and sickness insurance.

Section 4. Method of Disclosure of Required Information

All information required to be disclosed by these rules shall be set out conspicuously and in close conjunction with the statements to which such information relates or under appropriate captions of such prominence that it shall not be minimized, rendered obscure or presented in an ambiguous fashion or intermingled with the context of the advertisements so as to be confusing or misleading.

Section 5. Form and Content of Advertisements

A. The format and content of an advertisement of an accident or sickness insurance policy shall be sufficiently complete and clear to avoid deception or the capacity or tendency to mislead or deceive. Whether an advertisement has a capacity or tendency to mislead or deceive shall be determined by the Commissioner of Insurance from the overall impression that the advertisement may be reasonably expected to create upon a person of average education or intelligence, within the segment of the public to which it is directed.

B. Advertisements shall be truthful and not misleading in fact or in implication. Words or phrases, the meaning of which is clear only by implication or by familiarity with insurance terminology, shall not be used.

C. An insurer must clearly identify its accident and sickness insurance policy as an insurance policy. A policy trade name must be followed by the words "Insurance Policy" or similar words clearly identifying the fact that an insurance policy or health benefits product (in the case of health maintenance organizations, prepaid health plans and other direct service organizations) is being offered.

D. No insurer, agent, broker, producer, solicitor or other person shall solicit a resident of this State for the purchase of accident and sickness insurance in connection with or as the result of the use of advertisement by such person or any other persons, where the advertisement:

  (1) Contains any misleading representations or misrepresentations, or is otherwise untrue, deceptive or misleading with regard to the information imparted, the status, character or representative capacity of such person or the true purpose of the advertisement; or

  (2) Otherwise violates the provisions of these rules.

E. No insurer, agent, broker, producer, solicitor or other person shall solicit residents of this State for the purchase of accident and sickness insurance through the use of a true or fictitious name which is deceptive or misleading with regard to the status, character, or proprietary or representative capacity of such person or the true purpose of the advertisement.

Section 6. Advertisements of Benefits Payable, Losses Covered or Premiums Payable

A. Deceptive Words, Phrases or Illustrations Prohibited

  (1) No advertisement shall omit information or use words, phrases, statements, references or illustrations if the omission of such information or use of such words, phrases, statements, references or illustrations has the capacity, tendency or effect of misleading

or deceiving purchasers or prospective purchasers as to the nature or extent of any policy benefit payable, loss covered or premium payable. The fact that the policy offered is made available to a prospective insured for inspection prior to consummation of the sale or an offer is made to refund the premium if the purchaser is not satisfied, does not remedy misleading statements.

(2) No advertisement shall contain or use words or phrases such as "all," "full," "complete," "comprehensive," "unlimited," "up to," "as high as," "this policy will help fill some of the gaps that Medicare and your present insurance leave out," "the policy will help to replace your income," (when used to express loss of time benefits), or similar words and phrases, in a manner which exaggerates any benefits beyond the terms of the policy.

(3) An advertisement which also is an invitation to join an association, trust or discretionary group must solicit insurance coverage on a separate and distinct application which requires separate signatures for each application. The separate and distinct applications required need not be on a separate document or contained in a separate mailing. The insurance program must be presented so as not to mislead or deceive the prospective members that they are purchasing insurance as well as applying for membership, if that is the case.

(4) An advertisement shall not contain descriptions of policy limitations, exceptions or reductions, worded in a positive manner to imply that it is a benefit, such as describing a waiting period as a "benefit builder" or stating "even preexisting conditions are covered after two years." Words and phrases used in an advertisement to describe such policy limitations, exceptions and reductions shall fairly and accurately describe the negative features of such limitations, exceptions and reductions of the policy offered.

(5) An advertisement of accident and sickness insurance sold by direct response shall not state or imply that because "no insurance agent will call and no commissions will be paid to 'agents' that it is 'a low cost plan,'" or use other similar words or phrases because the cost of advertising and servicing such policies is a substantial cost in the marketing by direct response.

(6) No advertisement of a benefit for which payment is conditional upon confinement in a hospital or similar facility shall use words or phrases such as "tax-free," "extra cash," "extra income," "extra pay," or substantially similar words or phrases because such words and phrases have the capacity, tendency or effect of misleading the public into believing that the policy advertised will, in some way, enable them to make a profit from being hospitalized.

(7) No advertisement of a hospital or other similar facility confinement benefit shall advertise that the amount of the benefit is payable on a monthly or weekly basis when, in fact, the amount of the benefit payable is based upon a daily pro rata basis relating to the number of days of confinement unless such statements of such monthly or weekly benefit amounts are in juxtaposition with equally prominent statements of the benefit payable on a daily basis. The term "juxtaposition" means side by side or immediately above or below. When the policy contains a limit on the number of days of coverage provided, such limit must appear in the advertisement.

(8) No advertisement of a policy covering only one disease or a list of specified diseases shall imply coverage beyond the terms of the policy. Synonymous terms shall not be used to refer to any disease so as to imply broader coverage than is the fact.

APPENDIX D

(9) An advertisement for a policy providing benefits for specified illnesses only, such as cancer, or for specified accidents only, such as automobile accidents, shall clearly and conspicuously in prominent type state the limited nature of the policy. The statement shall be worded in language identical to or substantially similar to the following: "THIS IS A LIMITED POLICY," "THIS IS A CANCER ONLY POLICY," or "THIS IS AN AUTOMOBILE ACCIDENT ONLY POLICY."

B. Exceptions, Reductions and Limitations

(1) An advertisement which is an invitation to contract shall disclose those exceptions, reductions and limitations affecting the basic provisions of the policy.

(2) When a policy contains a waiting, elimination, probationary or similar time period between the effective date of the policy and the effective date of coverage under the policy or at a time period between the date a loss occurs and the date benefits begin to accrue for such loss, an advertisement which is subject to the requirements of the preceding paragraph shall disclose the existence of such periods.

(3) An advertisement shall not use the words "only," "just," "merely," "minimum," "necessary" or similar words or phrases to describe the applicability of any exceptions, reductions, limitations or exclusions such as: "This policy is subject to the following minimum exceptions and reductions."

C. Preexisting Conditions

(1) An advertisement which is an invitation to contract shall, in negative terms, disclose the extent to which any loss is not covered if the cause of such loss is traceable to a condition existing prior to the effective date of the policy. The use of the term "preexisting condition" without an appropriate definition or description shall not be used.

(2) When an accident and sickness insurance policy does not cover losses resulting from preexisting conditions, no advertisement of the policy shall state or imply that the applicant's physical condition or medical history will not affect the issuance of the policy or payment of a claim thereunder. This rule prohibits the use of the phrase "no medical examination required" and phrases of similar import, but does not prohibit explaining "automatic issue." If an insurer requires a medical examination for a specified policy, the advertisement if it is an invitation to contract shall disclose that a medical examination is required.

(3) When an advertisement contains an application form to be completed by the applicant and returned by mail, such application form shall contain a question or statement which reflects the preexisting condition provisions of the policy immediately preceding the blank space for the applicant's signature. For example, such an application form shall contain a question or statement substantially as follows:

Do you understand that this policy will not pay benefits during the first [insert number] year(s) after the issue date for a disease or physical condition which you now have or have had in the past?   YES

Or substantially the following statement:

I understand that the policy applied for will not pay benefits for any loss incurred during the first [insert number] year(s) after the issue date on account of disease or physical condition which I now have or have had in the past.

225

SUPPLEMENTAL HEALTH INSURANCE

Section 7. Necessity for Disclosing Policy Provisions Relating to Renewability, Cancellability and Termination

An advertisement which is an invitation to contract shall disclose the provisions relating to renewability, cancellability and termination and any modification of benefits, losses covered, or premiums because of age or for other reasons, in a manner which shall not minimize or render obscure the qualifying conditions.

Section 8. Testimonials or Endorsements by Third Parties

A. Testimonials and endorsements used in advertisements must be genuine, represent the current opinion of the author, be applicable to the policy advertised and be accurately reproduced. The insurer, in using a testimonial or endorsement, makes as its own all of the statements contained therein, and the advertisement, including such statement, is subject to all the provisions of these rules. When a testimonial or endorsement is used more than one year after it was originally given, a confirmation must be obtained.

B. A person shall be deemed a "spokesperson" if the person making the testimonial or endorsement:

(1) Has a financial interest in the insurer or a related entity as a stockholder, director, officer, employee or otherwise; or

(2) Has been formed by the insurer, is owned or controlled by the insurer, its employees, or the person or persons who own or control the insurer; or

(3) Has any person in a policy-making position who is affiliated with the insurer in any of the above described capacities; or

(4) Is in any way directly or indirectly compensated for making a testimonial or endorsement.

C. The fact of a financial interest or the proprietary or representative capacity of a spokesperson shall be disclosed in an advertisement and shall be accomplished in the introductory portion of the testimonial or endorsement in the same form and with equal prominence thereto. If a spokesperson is directly or indirectly compensated for making a testimonial or endorsement, such fact shall be disclosed in the advertisement by language substantially as follows: "Paid Endorsement." The requirement of this disclosure may be fulfilled by use of the phrase "Paid Endorsement" or words of similar import in a type style and size at least equal to that used for the spokesperson's name or the body of the testimonial or endorsement whichever is larger. In the case of television or radio advertising, the required disclosure must be accomplished in the introductory portion of the advertisement and must be given prominence.

D. The disclosure requirements of this rule shall not apply where the sole financial interest or compensation of a spokesperson, for all testimonials or endorsements made on behalf of the insurer, consists of the payment of union scale wages required by union rules, and if the payment is actually for such scale for TV or radio performances.

E. An advertisement shall not state or imply that an insurer or an accident and sickness insurance policy has been approved or endorsed by any individual, group of individuals, society, association or other organizations, unless such is the fact, and unless any proprietary relationship between an organization and the insurer is disclosed. If the entity making the endorsement or testimonial has been formed by the insurer or is owned or controlled by the insurer or the person or persons who own or control the insurer, such fact shall be disclosed

APPENDIX D

in the advertisement. If the insurer or an officer of the insurer formed or controls the association, or holds any policy-making position in the association, that fact must be disclosed.

F. When a testimonial refers to benefits received under an accident and sickness insurance policy, the specific claim data, including claim number, date of loss and other pertinent information shall be retained by the insurer for inspection for a period of four years or until the filing of the next regular report of examination of the insurer, whichever is the longer period of time. The use of testimonials which do not correctly reflect the present practices of the insurer or which are not applicable to the policy or benefit being advertised is not permissible.

Section 9. Use of Statistics

A. An advertisement relating to the dollar amounts of claims paid, the number of persons insured, or similar statistical information relating to any insurer or policy shall not use irrelevant facts, and shall not be used unless it accurately reflects all of the relevant facts. Such an advertisement shall not imply that such statistics are derived from the policy advertised unless such is the fact, and when applicable to other policies or plans shall specifically so state.

  (1) An advertisement shall specifically identify the accident and sickness insurance policy to which statistics relate and where statistics are given which are applicable to a different policy, it must be stated clearly that the data do not relate to the policy being advertised.

  (2) An advertisement using statistics which describe an insurer, such as assets, corporate structure, financial standing, age, product lines or relative position in the insurance business, may be irrelevant and, if used at all, must be used with extreme caution because of the potential for misleading the public. As a specific example, an advertisement for accident and sickness insurance which refers to the amount of life insurance which the company has in force or the amounts paid out in life insurance benefits is not permissible unless the advertisement clearly indicates the amount paid out for each line of insurance.

B. An advertisement shall not represent or imply that claim settlements by the insurer are "liberal" or "generous," or use words of similar import, or that claim settlements are or will be beyond the actual terms of the contract. An unusual amount paid for a unique claim for the policy advertised is misleading and shall not be used.

C. The source of any statistics used in an advertisement shall be identified in such advertisement.

Section 10. Identification of Plan or Number of Policies

A. When a choice of the amount of benefits is referred to, an advertisement which is an invitation to contract shall disclose that the amount of benefits provided depends upon the plan selected and that the premium will vary with the amount of the benefits selected.

B. When an advertisement which is an invitation to contract refers to various benefits which may be contained in two or more policies, other than group master policies, the advertisement shall disclose that such benefits are provided only though a combination of such policies.

Section 11. Disparaging Comparisons and Statements

An advertisement shall not directly or indirectly make unfair or incomplete comparisons of policies or benefits or comparisons of non-comparable policies of other insurers, and shall not disparage competitors, their policies, services or business methods, and shall not disparage or unfairly minimize competing methods of marketing insurance.

A. An advertisement shall not contain statements such as "no red tape" or "here is all you do to receive benefits."

B. Advertisements which state or imply that competing insurance coverages customarily contain certain exceptions, reductions or limitations not contained in the advertised policies are unacceptable unless such exceptions, reductions or limitations are contained in a substantial majority of such competing coverages.

C. Advertisements which state or imply that an insurer's premiums are lower or that its loss ratios are higher because its organizational structure differs from that of competing insurers are unacceptable.

Section 12. Jurisdictional Licensing and Status of Insurer

A. An advertisement which is intended to be seen or heard beyond the limits of the jurisdiction in which the insurer is licensed shall not imply licensing beyond those limits.

B. An advertisement shall not create the impression directly or indirectly that the insurer, its financial condition or status, or the payment of its claims, or the merits, desirability, or advisability of its policy forms or kinds or plans of insurance are approved, endorsed or accredited by any division or agency of this State or the United States Government.

C. An advertisement shall not imply that approval, endorsement or accreditation of policy forms or advertising has been granted by any division or agency of the state or federal government. "Approval" of either policy forms or advertising shall not be used by an insurer to imply or state that a governmental agency has endorsed or recommended the insurer, its policies, advertising or its financial condition.

Section 13. Identity of Insurer

A. The name of the actual insurer shall be stated in all of its advertisements. The form number or numbers of the policy advertised shall be stated in an advertisement which is an invitation to contract. An advertisement shall not use a trade name, any insurance group designation, name of the parent company of the insurer, name of a particular division of the insurer, service mark, slogan, symbol or other device which without disclosing the name of the actual insurer would have the capacity and tendency to mislead or deceive as to the true identity of the insurer.

B. No advertisement shall use any combination of words, symbols, or physical materials which by their content, phraseology, shape, color or other characteristics are so similar to combination of words, symbols or physical materials used by agencies of the federal government or of this State, or otherwise appear to be of such a nature that it tends to confuse or mislead prospective insureds into believing that the solicitation is in some manner connected with an agency of the municipal, state or federal government.

C. Advertisements, envelopes or stationery which employ words, letters, initials, symbols or other devices which are so similar to those used in governmental agencies or by other insurers are not permitted if they may lead the public to believe:

(1) That the advertised coverages are somehow provided by or are endorsed by such governmental agencies or such other insurers;

(2) That the advertiser is the same as, is connected with or is endorsed by such governmental agencies or such other insurers.

D. No advertisement shall use the name of a state or political subdivision thereof in a policy name or description.

E. No advertisement in the form of envelopes or stationery of any kind may use any name, service mark, slogan, symbol or any device in such a manner that implies that the insurer or the policy advertised, or that any agent who may call upon the consumer in response to the advertisement is connected with a governmental agency, such as the Social Security Administration.

F. No advertisement may incorporate the word "Medicare" in the title of the plan or policy being advertised unless, wherever it appears, said word is qualified by language differentiating it from Medicare. Such an advertisement, however, shall not use the phrase "[   ] Medicare Department of the [   ] Insurance Company," or language of similar import.

G. No advertisement may imply that the reader may lose a right or privilege or benefit under federal, state or local law if he fails to respond to the advertisement.

H. The use of letters, initials, or symbols of the corporate name or trademark that would have the tendency or capacity to mislead or deceive the public as to the true identity of the insurer is prohibited unless the true, correct and complete name of the insurer is in close conjunction and in the same size type as the letters, initials or symbols of the corporate name or trademark.

I. The use of the name of an agency or "[   ] Underwriters" or "[   ] Plan" in type, size and location so as to have the capacity and tendency to mislead or deceive as to the true identity of the insurer is prohibited.

J. The use of an address so as to mislead or deceive as to true identity of the insurer, its location or licensing status is prohibited.

K. No insurer may use, in the trade name of its insurance policy, any terminology or words so similar to the name of a governmental agency or governmental program as to have the tendency to confuse, deceive or mislead the prospective purchaser.

L. All advertisements used by agents, producers, brokers or solicitors of an insurer must have prior written approval of the insurer before they may be used.

M. An agent who makes contact with a consumer, as a result of acquiring that consumer's name from a lead-generating device, must disclose such fact in the initial contact with the consumer.

Section 14. Group or Quasi-Group Implications

A. An advertisement of a particular policy shall not state or imply that prospective insureds become group or quasi-group members covered under a group policy and as such enjoy special rates or underwriting privileges, unless such is the fact.

B. This rule prohibits the solicitations of a particular class, such as governmental employees, by use of advertisements which state or imply that their occupational status entitles them to reduced rates on a group or other basis when, in fact, the policy being advertised is sold only on an individual basis at regular rates.

Section 15. Introductory, Initial or Special Offers

A. (1) An advertisement of an individual policy shall not directly or by implication represent that a contract or combination of contracts is an introductory, initial or special offer, or that applicants will receive substantial advantages not available at a later date, or that the offer is available only to a specified group of individuals, unless such is the fact. An advertisement shall not contain phrases describing an enrollment period as "special," "limited," or similar words or phrases when the insurer uses such enrollment periods as the usual method of advertising accident and sickness insurance.

(2) An enrollment period during which a particular insurance product may be purchased on an individual basis shall not be offered within this State unless there has been a lapse of not less than [insert number] months between the close of the immediately preceding enrollment period for the same product and the opening of the new enrollment period. The advertisement shall indicate the date by which the applicant must mail the application, which shall be not less than ten days and not more than forty days from the date that such enrollment period is advertised for the first time. This rule applies to all advertising media, i.e., mail, newspapers, radio, television, magazines and periodicals, by any one insurer. It is inapplicable to solicitations of employees or members of a particular group or association which otherwise would be eligible under specific provisions of the Insurance Code for group, blanket or franchise insurance. The phrase "any one insurer" includes all the affiliated companies of a group of insurance companies under common management or control.

NOTE: The number of months was left blank in this rule because several states currently permit six months, several states allow three months, and other states currently prohibit such periods of enrollment. Whether such enrollment periods should be permissible and the period of time between enrollment are items on which each state should make its own decision. Each state should modify the time limit in this guideline to comply with the rule adopted by the particular state.

(3) This rule prohibits any statement or implication to the effect that only a specific number of policies will be sold, or that a time is fixed for the discontinuance of the sale of the particular policy advertised because of special advantages available in the policy, unless such is the fact.

(4) The phrase "a particular insurance product" in Paragraph (2) of this section means an insurance policy which provides substantially different benefits than those contained in any other policy. Different terms of renewability; an increase or decrease in the dollar amounts of benefits; an increase or decrease in any elimination period or waiting period from those available during an enrollment period for another policy shall not be sufficient to constitute the product being offered as a different product eligible for concurrent or overlapping enrollment periods.

B. An advertisement shall not offer a policy which utilizes a reduced initial premium rate in a manner which overemphasizes the availability and the amount of the initial reduced premium. When an insurer charges an initial premium that differs in amount from the amount of the renewal premium payable on the same mode, the advertisement shall not display the amount of the reduced initial premium either more frequently or more prominently than the renewal premium, and both the initial reduced premium and the renewal premium must be stated in juxtaposition in each portion of the advertisement where the initial reduced premium appears.

NOTE: Some states prohibit a reduced initial premium. Section 15B does not imply that the states which prohibit such initial premium are not in conformity with the NAIC Rules. This item is indicated in the rule as an item to be decided on a state-by-state basis.

C. Special awards, such as a "safe drivers' award" shall not be used in connection with advertisements of accident and sickness insurance.

Section 16. Statements About an Insurer

An advertisement shall not contain statements which are untrue in fact, or by implication misleading, with respect to the assets, corporate structure, financial standing, age or relative position of the insurer in the insurance business. An advertisement shall not contain a recommendation by any commercial rating system unless it clearly indicates the purpose of the recommendation and the limitations of the scope and extent of the recommendations.

Section 17. Enforcement Procedures

A. Advertising File. Each insurer shall maintain at its home or principal office a complete file containing every printed, published or prepared advertisement of its individual policies and typical printed, published or prepared advertisements of its blanket, franchise and group policies hereafter disseminated in this or any other state, whether or not licensed in such other state, with a notation attached to each such advertisement which shall indicate the manner and extent of distribution and the form number of any policy advertised. Such file shall be subject to regular and periodical inspection by this Department. All such advertisements shall be maintained in said file for a period of either four years or until the filing of the next regular report on examination of the insurer, whichever is the longer period of time.

B. Certificate of Compliance. Each insurer required to file an Annual Statement which is now or which hereafter becomes subject to the provisions of these rules must file with this Department, with its annual statement, a certificate of compliance executed by an authorized officer of the insurer wherein it is stated that, to the best of his knowledge, information and belief, the advertisements which were disseminated by the insurer during the preceding statement year complied or were made to comply in all respects with the provisions of these rules and the insurance laws of this State as implemented and interpreted by these rules.

NOTE: Where the rules were adopted on other than January 1 of the year, the required certification that all advertisements used in the preceding annual statement year complied with these rules cannot be given. The respective insurance departments should consider remedying the problem in the Certificate of Compliance used for the calendar year in which the rules were adopted.

Section 18. Severability Provision

If any section or portion of a section of these rules, or the applicability thereof to any person or circumstance is held invalid by a court, the remainder of the rules, or the applicability of such provision to other persons or circumstances, shall not be affected thereby.

Section 19. Filing for Prior Review

The Commissioner may, at his discretion, require the filing with the Department, for review prior to use, of any accident and sickness insurance advertising material. Such advertising material must be filed by the insurer with the Department not less than thirty days prior to the date the insurer desires to use the advertisement.

Appendix

**INTERPRETIVE GUIDELINES
FOR RULES GOVERNING ADVERTISEMENTS
OF ACCIDENT AND SICKNESS
INSURANCE**

Guideline 1.

Disclosure is one of the principal objectives of these rules and this section states specifically that the rules shall assure "truthful and adequate disclosure of all material and relevant information." These rules specifically prohibit some previous advertising techniques.

Guideline 2-A.

These rules apply to any "advertisement" as that term is defined in Section 3, Subsections A, H, I and J unless otherwise specified in the rules.

These rules apply to group and blanket as well as individual accident and sickness insurance. Certain distinctions, however, are applicable to these categories. Among them is the level of conversance with insurance, a factor which is covered by Section 5A of the rules.

Guideline 3-A.

The scope of the term "advertisement" extends to the use of all media for communications to the general public, to the use of all media for communications to specific members of the general public, and to the use of all media for communications by agents, brokers, producers and solicitors.

Guideline 3-B.

In Section 3B, the language "except disability, waiver of premium and double indemnity benefits included in life insurance and annuity contracts" means except disability, waiver of premium and double indemnity benefits included in life insurance, endowment or annuity contracts or contracts supplemental thereto which contain only such provisions which: (1) provide additional benefits in case of death or dismemberment or loss of sight by accident or as (2) operate to safeguard such contracts against lapse or to give a special surrender value or special benefit or an annuity in the event that the insured or annuitant shall become totally and permanently disabled as defined by the contract or supplemental contract.

Guideline 3-I.

1. A "brief description of coverage" in an invitation to inquire must be limited to a brief description of the loss for which benefits are payable but may contain:

    (a) The dollar amount of benefits payable; and/or

    (b) The period of time during which benefits are payable.

2. An invitation to inquire may not refer to cost.

3. As with all accident and sickness insurance advertisements, an invitation to inquire must not:

(a) Employ devices which are designed to create undue anxiety;

(b) Exaggerate the value of the benefits available under the advertised policy;

(c) Otherwise violate the provisions of these rules.

Guideline 4.

The rule permits the use of either of the following methods of disclosure:

1. The first method provides for the disclosure of exceptions, limitations, reductions and other restrictions conspicuously and in close conjunction with the statements to which such information relates. This may be accomplished by disclosure in the description of the related benefits or in a paragraph set out in close conjunction with the description of policy benefits.
2. The second method provides for the disclosure of exceptions, limitations, reductions and other restrictions not in conjunction with the provisions describing policy benefits but under appropriate captions of such prominence that the information shall not be minimized, rendered obscure or otherwise made to appear unimportant. The phrase "under appropriate captions" means that the title must be accurately descriptive of the captioned material. Appropriate captions include the following: "Exceptions," "Exclusions," "Conditions Not Covered," and "Exceptions and Reductions." The use of captions such as, or similar to, the following are not acceptable because they do not provide adequate notice of the significance of the material: "Extent of Coverage," "Only these Exclusions," or "Minimum Limitations."

In considering whether an advertisement complies with the disclosure requirements of this rule, the rule must be applied in conjunction with the form and content standards contained in Section 5.

Guideline 5-A.

The rule must be applied in conjunction with Sections 1 and 4 of the rules. This rule refers specifically to "format and content" of the advertisement and the "overall" impression created by the advertisement. This involves factors such as, but not limited to, the size, color and prominence of type used to describe benefits. The word "format" means the arrangement of the text and the captions.

The rule requires distinctly different advertisements for publication in newspapers or magazines of general circulation as compared to scholarly, technical or business journals and newspapers. Where an advertisement consists of more than one piece of material, each piece of material must, independent of all other pieces of material, conform to the disclosure requirements of the rule.

Guideline 5-B.

The rule prohibits the use of incomplete statements and words or phrases which have the tendency or capacity to mislead or deceive because of the reader's unfamiliarity with insurance terminology. Therefore, words, phrases and illustrations used in an advertisement must be clear and unambiguous and, if the advertisement uses insurance terminology, sufficient description of a word, phrase or illustration shall be provided by definition or description in the context of the advertisement. As implied in Guideline 5-A, distinctly different levels of comprehension of the subscribers of various publications may be anticipated.

SUPPLEMENTAL HEALTH INSURANCE

Guideline 6-A(1).

The following examples are illustrations of the prohibitions created by the rule:

1. An advertisement which describes any benefits that vary by age must disclose that fact.

2. An advertisement which uses a phrase such as "no age limit," if benefits or premiums vary by age or if age is an underwriting factor, must disclose that fact.

3. Advertisements, applications, requests for additional information and similar materials are unacceptable if they state or imply that the recipient has been individually selected to be offered insurance or has had his eligibility for such insurance individually determined in advance when the advertisement is directed to all persons in a group or to all persons whose names appear on a mailing list.

4. Advertisements which indicate that a particular coverage or policy is exclusively for "preferred risks" or a particular segment of the population or that a particular segment of the population are acceptable risks, when such distinctions are not maintained in the issuance of policies, are not acceptable.

5. Advertisements for group or franchise group plans which provide a common benefit or a common combination of benefits shall not imply that the insurance coverage is tailored or designed specifically for that group, unless such is the fact.

6. It is unacceptable to use terms such as "enroll" or "join" to imply group or blanket insurance coverage when such is not the fact.

7. Any advertisement which contains statements such as "anyone can apply," or "anyone can join," other than with respect to a guaranteed issue policy for which administrative procedures exist to assure that the policy is issued within a reasonable period of time after the application is received by the insurer.

8. An advertisement which states or implies immediate coverage of a policy is unacceptable unless suitable administrative procedures exist so that the policy is issued within fifteen working days after the application is received by the insurer.

9. Any advertisement which contains statements such as "here is all you do to apply," "simply" or "merely" to refer to the act of applying for a policy which is not a guaranteed issue policy is unacceptable unless it refers to the fact that the application is subject to acceptance or approval by the insurer.

10. Applications, request forms for additional information and similar related materials are unacceptable if they resemble paper currency, bonds, stock certificates, etc.; or use any name, service mark, slogan, symbol or any device in such a manner that implies that the insurer or the policy advertised is connected with a government agency, such as the Social Security Administration or the Department of Health and Human Services.

11. No advertisement shall employ devices which are designed to create undue fear or anxiety in the minds of those to whom they are directed. Unacceptable examples of such devices are:

    (a) The use of phrases such as "cancer kills somebody every two minutes" and "total number of accidents" without reference to the total population from which such statistics are drawn. (As an example of a permissible device, data prepared by the American Cancer Society are acceptable provided their source is noted and they are not overemphasized);

APPENDIX D

(b) The use of phrases such as "the finest kind of treatment," implying that such treatment would be unavailable without insurance;

(c) The reproduction of newspaper articles, etc., containing irrelevant facts and figures;

(d) The use of illustrations which unduly emphasize automobile accidents, cripples or persons confined in beds who are in obvious distress or receiving hospital or medical bills or persons being evicted from their homes due to their hospital bills;

(e) The use of phrases such as "financial disaster," "financial distress," "financial shock," or other phrases implying that financial ruin is likely without insurance, where used in an advertisement which comes within Section 6A(9) relating to policies covering specified illnesses or specified accidents only.

12. An advertisement which uses the word "plan" without identifying it as an accident and sickness insurance policy is not permissible.

13. An advertisement which implies in any manner that the prospective insured may realize a profit from obtaining hospital, medical or surgical insurance coverage is not permissible.

14. An advertisement shall not state or imply by word, phrase or illustration that the benefits being offered will supplement any other insurance policy, insurance-type concept, or governmental plan if such is not the fact.

15. An advertisement of a hospital or other similar facility confinement benefit that makes reference to the benefit being paid directly to the policyholder is misleading unless, in making such a reference, the advertisement includes a statement that the benefits may be paid directly to the hospital or other health care facility if an assignment of benefits is made by the policyholder. An advertisement of medical and surgical expense benefits shall comply with this rule in regard to the disclosure of assignments of benefits to providers of services. Phrases such as "you collect," "you get paid," "pays you," or other words or phrases of similar import are acceptable so long as the advertisement indicates that it is payable to the insured or someone designated by the insured.

16. An advertisement which refers to "hospitalization for injury or sickness" omitting the word "covered" when the policy excludes certain sicknesses or injuries, or which refers to "whenever you are hospitalized" or "while you are confined in the hospital" omitting the phrase "for covered injury or sickness," if the policy excludes certain injuries or sickness is unacceptable. Continued reference to "covered injury or sickness" is not necessary where this fact has been prominently disclosed in the advertisement and where the description of sicknesses or injuries not covered are prominently set forth.

17. Advertisements which state that benefits are provided when "you go to the hospital" are unacceptable unless the advertisement clearly sets forth the extent of the coverage.

18. An advertisement which fails to disclose that the definition of "hospital" does not include a nursing home, convalescent home or extended care facility, as the case may be, is unacceptable.

19. An advertisement which fails to disclose any waiting or elimination periods for specific benefits is unacceptable.

20. An advertisement for a limited policy, or hospital indemnity policy, or a plan of insurance which covers only certain causes of loss (such as dread disease) or which covers only a certain type of loss (such as hospital confinement) is unacceptable if:

(a) The advertisement refers to a total benefit maximum limit payable under the policy in any headline, lead-in or caption without also in the same headline, lead-in or caption specifying the applicable daily limits and other internal limits;

(b) The advertisement states any total benefit limit without stating the periodic benefit payment, if any, and the length of time the periodic benefit would be payable to reach the total benefit limit;

(c) The advertisement prominently displays a total benefit limit which would not, as a general rule, be payable under an average claim.

21. Advertisements which emphasize total amounts payable under hospital, medical or surgical accident and sickness insurance coverage or other benefits in a policy, such as benefits for private duty nursing, are unacceptable unless the actual amounts payable per day for such indemnity or benefits are stated.

22. Examples of benefits payable under a policy shall not disclose only maximum benefits unless such maximum benefits are paid for loss from common and probable illnesses or accidents rather than exceptional or rare illnesses or accidents or periods of confinement for such exceptional or rare accidents or illnesses.

23. When a range of benefit levels is set forth in an advertisement, it must be made clear that the insured will receive only the benefit level written or printed in the policy selected and issued. Language which implies that the insured may select the benefit level at the time of filing claims is unacceptable.

24. Language which implies that the amount of benefits payable under a loss-of-time policy may be increased at the time of claim or disability according to the needs of the insured is unacceptable.

25. An advertisement for loss-of-time coverage which is an invitation to contract which sets forth a range of amounts of benefit levels is unacceptable unless it also states that eligibility for the benefits is based upon condition of health, income or other economic conditions, or other underwriting standards of the insurer if such is the fact.

26. The term "confining sickness" is an abbreviated expression and must be explained in an advertisement containing the term. Such an explanation might be as follows: "Benefits are payable for total disability due to confining sickness only so long as the insured is necessarily confined indoors." Captions such as "Lifetime Sickness Benefits" or "Five-Year Sickness Benefits" are incomplete if such benefits are subject to confinement requirements. When sickness benefits are subject to confinement requirements, captions such as "Lifetime House Confining Sickness Benefits" or "Five-Year House Confining Sickness Benefits" would be permissible.

27. Advertisements for policies whose premiums are modest because of their limited coverage or limited amount of benefits shall not describe premiums as "low," "low cost," "budget" or use qualifying words of similar import. This rule also prohibits the use of words such as "only" and "just" in conjunction with statements of premium amounts when used to imply a bargain.

28. Advertisements which state or imply that premiums will not be changed in the future are not acceptable unless the advertised policies so provide.

29. An advertisement which does not require the premium to accompany the application must not overemphasize that fact and must make the effective date of that coverage clear.

APPENDIX D

30. An advertisement which exaggerates the effects of statutorily mandated benefits or required policy provisions or which implies that such provisions are unique to the advertised policy is unacceptable. For example, the phrase, "Money Back Guarantee" is an exaggerated description of the "free look" right to examine the policy and is not acceptable.

31. An advertisement which implies that a common type of policy or a combination of common benefits is "new," "unique," "a bonus," "a breakthrough," or is otherwise unusual is unacceptable. Also, the addition of a novel method of premium payment to an otherwise common plan of insurance does not render it "new."

32. An advertisement which is an invitation to contract which fails to disclose the amount of any deductible and/or the percentage of any co-insurance factor is not acceptable.

33. An advertisement which fails to state clearly the type of insurance coverage being offered is not acceptable.

34. Language which states or implies that each member under a "family" contract is covered as to the maximum benefits advertised, where such is not the fact, is not acceptable.

35. The importance of diseases rarely or seldom found in the class of persons to whom the policy is offered shall not be exaggerated in an advertisement.

36. A television, radio, mail or newspaper advertisement or lead-generating device which is designed to produce leads either by use of a coupon a request to write or to call the company or a subsequent advertisement prior to contact must include information disclosing that an agent may contact the applicant if such is the fact.

37. Phrases or devices which unduly excite fear of dependence upon relatives or charity are unacceptable. Phrases or devices which imply that long sicknesses or hospital stays are common among the elderly are unacceptable.

Guideline 6-A(2).

This rule recognizes that certain words and phrases in advertising may have a tendency to mislead the public as to the extent of benefits under an advertised policy. Consequently, such terms (and those specified in the rule do not represent a comprehensive list but only examples) must be used with caution to avoid any tendency to exaggerate benefits and must not be used unless the statement is literally true in every instance. The use of the following phrases based on such terms or having the same effect must be similarly restricted: "pays hospital, surgical, etc., bills," "pays dollars to offset the cost of medical care," "safeguards your standard of living," "pays full coverage," "pays complete coverage," "pays for financial needs," "provides for replacement of your lost paycheck," "replaces income" or "emergency paycheck." Other phrases may or may not be acceptable depending upon the nature of the coverage being advertised. For example, the phrase "this policy will help to replace your income" is acceptable in advertising for loss-of-time coverage but is unacceptable in advertising for hospital confinement (including "hospital indemnity") coverage.

This rule also prohibits words or phrases which exaggerate the effect of benefit payments on the insured's general well-being, such as "worry-free savings plan," "guaranteed savings," "financial peace of mind," and "you will never have to worry about hospital bills again."

Guideline 6-A(4).

Negative features must be accurately set forth. Any limitation on benefits precluding preexisting conditions also must be restated under a caption concerning exclusions or limitations, notwithstanding that the preexisting condition exclusion has been disclosed elsewhere in the advertisement. (See Guideline 6-C for additional comments on preexisting conditions.)

Guideline 6-A(5).

This rule should be applied in conjunction with Section 11. Phrases such as "we cut costs to the bone" or "we deal direct with you so our costs are lower" shall not be used.

Guideline 6-A(6).

The words, phrases, illustrations and concepts listed are illustrations of the words, phrases, illustrations and concepts prohibited by the rule which creates the impression of a profit or gain to be realized by the insured when hospitalized.

Illustrations which depict paper currency or checks showing an amount payable are deceptive and misleading and are not permissible.

A hospital indemnity advertisement shall not include language such as "pay for a trip to Florida," "buy a new television," or otherwise imply that the insured will make a profit on hospitalization.

An advertisement which uses words such as "extra," "special," or "added" to describe any benefit in the policy is unacceptable.

Although the rule prohibits the use of the phrase "tax free," it does not prohibit the use of complete and accurate terminology explaining the Internal Revenue Service rules applicable to the taxation of accident and sickness benefits. The IRS rules provide that the premiums paid for and the benefits received from hospital indemnity policies are subject to the same rules as loss of time premiums and benefits and are not afforded the same favorable tax treatment as premiums for expense incurred hospital, medical and surgical benefit coverages. (Rev. Rul. 68-451 and Rev. Rul. 69-154.) Prominence either by caption, lead-in, bold-face or large type shall not be given in any manner to any statements relating to the tax status of such benefits.

Guideline 6-B(1).

An advertisement which is an invitation to contract as defined in Section 3-J must recite the exceptions, reductions, and limitations as required by the rule and in a manner consistent with Section 4.

If an exception, reduction or limitation is important enough to use in a policy, it is of sufficient importance that its existence in the policy should be referred to in the advertisement regardless of whether it may also be the subject matter of a provision of the Uniform Individual Accident and Sickness Provision Law.

Some advertisements disclose exceptions, reductions and limitations as required, but the advertisement is so lengthy as to obscure the disclosure. Where the length of an advertisement has this effect, special emphasis must be given by changing the format to show the restrictions in a manner which does not minimize, render obscure or otherwise make them appear unimportant.

Guideline 6-B(2).

The rule imposes the same disclosure standards as the preceding paragraph with respect to policy provisions providing for waiting, elimination, probationary or similar time periods between the effective date of the policy and the effective date of coverage under the policy or at a time period

APPENDIX D

between the date a loss occurs and the date benefits begin to accrue for such loss. The guideline for Subsection 6B(1) is equally applicable to this subsection. Where a policy has waiting, elimination, probationary or other such time periods, such provisions must be stated in negative terms. This requirement is comparable to that contemplated in Section 6A(4) as to exceptions, reductions and limitations.

Guideline 6-B(3).

The rule is similar to Section 6A(4) and requires a fair and accurate description of exceptions, limitations and reductions in a manner which does not minimize, render obscure or otherwise make them appear unimportant.

Advertisements must state exceptions, limitations and reductions in the negative and must not understate any exception, limitation or reduction or qualify any exception, limitation or reduction to emphasize coverage described elsewhere (e.g., "Does not pay for [insert exception, limitation or reduction], however, Medicare pays this" is not acceptable, nor is "Does not pay for the first four days in hospital for sickness, but pays for accident from first day"). (Underscoring indicates the manner in which statements are sometimes emphasized.)

Guideline 6-C(1).

The rule imposes the same disclosure standards with respect to preexisting conditions provisions as noted in Guideline 6-B(1). The comments under that guideline are equally applicable to this subsection of the rules since the preexisting conditions provision is an exception under the rules.

This rule implements the objective of Section 6A(3) by requiring in negative terms a description of the effect of a preexisting condition exclusion because such an exclusion is a restriction on coverage. The subdivision also prohibits the use of the phrase "preexisting condition" without an appropriate definition or description of the term and prohibits stating a reduction in the statutory time limit (such as a reduction from three years to two years or to one year) as an affirmative benefit. The words "appropriate definition or description" mean that the term "preexisting condition" must be defined as it is used by the company's claims department.

Guideline 6-C(2).

The phrase "no health questions" or words of similar import shall not be used if the policy excludes preexisting conditions.

Use of a phrase such as "guaranteed issue" or "automatic issue," if the policy excludes preexisting conditions for a certain period, must be accompanied by a statement disclosing that fact in a manner which does not minimize, render obscure, or otherwise make it appear unimportant and is otherwise consistent with Section 4.

Guideline 6-C(3).

Some states require approval of the application even when the application is not attached to the policy when issued. This rule does not change such a requirement. The text of this guideline should be modified to reflect the rule applicable in the particular state.

Guideline 7.

This rule imposes the same disclosure standards with respect to policy provisions relating to renewability, cancellability and termination, modification of benefits, losses or premiums because of age or otherwise as stated in Guideline 6-B(1). The comments in that guideline are equally applicable to this section.

Advertisements of cancellable accident and sickness insurance policies must state that the contract is cancellable or renewable at the option of the company as the case may be. With respect to noncancellable policies and guaranteed renewable policies, the policy provisions, with respect to renewability, must be set forth and defined where appropriate. For example the following represent illustrations: A policy which is cancellable shall be advertised in a manner similar to "This policy can be cancelled by the company at any time." A policy which is renewable at the option of the insurance company shall be advertised in a manner to "This policy is renewable at the option of the company" or "The company has the right to refuse renewal of this policy" or "Renewable at the option of the insurer." Advertisements of such policies must indicate that the insurer has the right to increase premium rates. With respect to non-cancellable policies and guaranteed renewable policies, the rule requires a summary of the policy provisions with respect to renewability must be set forth and defined where appropriate. The disclosure of provisions relating to renewability requires the use of language such as "non-cancellable," "non-cancellable and guaranteed renewable," or "guaranteed renewable." Unless otherwise modified by law or regulation in an individual state, the use of those terms and the definitions provided shall be consistent with the definitions of those terms adopted by the National Association of Insurance Commissioners (See 1960 NAIC Proceedings I 153).

The rule also requires a statement of the qualifying conditions which constitute limitations on the permanent nature of the coverage. These customarily fall into three categories: (1) age limits, (2) reservation of a right to increase premiums, and (3) the establishment of aggregate limits. For example, "non-cancellable and guaranteed renewable" does not fulfill the requirement of the rule if the policy contains a terminal age of sixty-five. In such a case, a proper statement would be "non-cancellable and guaranteed renewable to age sixty-five". If a guaranteed renewable policy reserves the right to increase premiums, the statement must be expanded into language similar to "guaranteed renewable to age sixty-five but the company reserves the right to increase premium rates on a class basis." If the contract contains an aggregate limit after which no further benefits are payable, the above statement must be amplified with the phrase "subject to a maximum aggregate amount of $50,000" or similar language. A policy may have one or more of the three basic limitations and an advertisement must describe each of those which the policy contains. Over fifty percent of new individual policy issues are guaranteed renewable; therefore, the fact that a policy is guaranteed renewable shall not be exaggerated.

This rule also requires the disclosure of any modification of benefits or losses covered because of age or for other reasons. Provisions for reduction of benefits at stated ages must be set forth. For example, a policy may contain a provision which reduces benefits fifty percent after age sixty although it is renewable to age sixty-five. Such a reduction would have to be set forth. Also, a provision for the elimination of certain hazards at any specific ages or after the policy has been in force for a specified time would have to be set forth.

An advertisement for a policy which provides for step-rated premium rates based upon the policy year or the insured's attained age must disclose such rate increases and the times or ages at which such premiums increase.

This rule requires that the qualifying conditions of renewability must be disclosed in a manner which does not minimize or render obscure the qualifying conditions of renewal.

Guideline 8-A.

The rule must be applied in conjunction with Section 9 and requires that all such statements must be genuine and not fictitious. Under the rule, the manufacturing, substantive editing or "doctoring up" of a testimonial is clearly prohibited as being false and misleading to the insurance-buying public. However, language which would be unacceptable under these rules must be edited out of a testimonial.

Guideline 8-B.

Reimbursement for substantial travel and entertainment expenses is also required to be disclosed; however, union scale wages required by union rules are not required to be disclosed. Travel away from the home of the person giving the testimonial or endorsement to a distant location involving transportation expenses, lodging expenses or expenses for meals constitutes payment and must be reflected as a paid endorsement.

Guideline 8-C.

The rule requires both that approval or endorsement of a policy by an individual, group of individuals, society, association, or other organization be factual and that any proprietary relationship between the sponsoring or endorsing organization and the insurer be disclosed. For example, if the dividend under an association group case is payable to the association, disclosure of that fact is required. Also, if the insurer or an officer of the insurer formed or controls the association, that fact must be disclosed. This guideline also applies to Section 8E.

Guideline 9-A.

This rule prohibits the use of statistics in a manner which is misleading and deceptive. This rule requires the disclosure of all relevant facts and prohibits the use of irrelevant facts.

An advertisement which states the dollar amount of claims paid must also indicate the period over which such claims have been paid.

If the term "loss ratio" is used, it shall be properly explained in the context of the advertisement and, unless the state has issued a regulation otherwise defining the term, it shall be calculated on the basis of premiums earned to losses incurred and shall not be on a yearly run-off basis.

Guideline 9-C.

The rule does not require that statistics for a state be used since such statistics as hospital charges and average stays may vary from state to state. When nationwide statistics are used such fact should be noted as such unless the statistics on the particular point are substantially the same in a state to which the advertisement is directed. Statistics may be used only if they are credible.

Guideline 11.

The rule prohibits disparaging, unfair or incomplete comparisons of policies or benefits which would have a tendency to deceive or mislead the public. The rule does not preclude the use of comparisons by health maintenance organizations, prepaid health plans and other direct service organizations which describe the difference between their prepaid health benefits coverage and indemnity insurance coverage.

Guideline 12-A.

The rule prohibits advertisements which imply that an insurer is licensed beyond the limits of those jurisdictions where it is actually licensed. An advertisement which contains testimonials from persons who reside in a state in which the insurer is not licensed or which refers to claims of persons residing in states in which the insurer is not licensed implies licensing in those states and therefore is in violation of this rule unless the advertisement states that the insurer is not licensed in those states.

Guideline 12-B.

Although the rule permits a reference to an insurer being licensed in a state where the advertisement appears, it does not allow exaggeration of the fact of such licensing nor does it permit the suggestion that competing insurers may not be so licensed because, in most states, an insurer must be licensed in the state to which it directs its advertising.

Terms such as "official," or words of similar import, used to describe any policy or application form are not permissible because of the potential for deceiving or misleading the public.

Guideline 13.

The rule recognizes the existence of holding companies. The requirement that the advertisement refer to the policy form number is applicable only to advertisements of individual and franchise policies that are invitations to contract.

Guideline 14.

The rule prohibits the use of representations to any segment of the population that a particular policy or coverage is available only to that or similar segments of the population as preferred risks when actually such policy or coverage is available to members of the public at large at the same rates. The rule prohibits an advertisement labeled "Now for Readers of X Magazine."

Guideline 15-A(1).

The rule prohibits advertising representing that a product is offered on an introductory, initial, special offer basis or otherwise which (1) will not be available later; or (2) is available only to certain individuals, unless such is the fact. This rule prohibits the repetitive use of such advertisements. Where an insurer uses enrollment periods as the usual method of advertising these policies, the rule prohibits describing an enrollment period as a special opportunity or offer for the applicant.

Guideline 15-A(2).

The rule restricts the repetitive use of enrollment periods. The requirement of reasonable closing dates and waiting periods between enrollment periods was adopted to eliminate the abuses which formerly existed. The rule does not limit just the use of enrollment periods. It requires that a particular insurance product offered in an enrollment period through any advertising media, including the prepared presentations of agents, cannot be offered again in the entire state until [insert number] months from the close of the enrollment period have expired. Thus, an insurer must choose whether to use enrollment periods or open enrollment for a product. (See Section 15A(4) for definitions of "a particular insurance product.")

The rule does not prohibit multiple advertising during an enrollment period through any and all media published or transmitted within this state as long as the enrollment periods for all such advertisements have the same expiration date.

The rule does not prohibit the solicitation of members of a group or association for the same product even though there has not been a lapse of [insert number] months since the close of a preceding enrollment period which was open to the general public for the same product.

The rule does not require separation by [insert number] months of enrollment periods for the same insurance product in this State if the advertising material is directed by an admitted insurer to persons by direct mail on the basis that a common relationship exists with an entity, such as a bank and its depositors, a department store to its charge account customers or an oil company to its credit card holders, and more than one of such organizations is sponsoring such insurance product at different times if providing such insurance under such a method is not otherwise prohibited by law; provided, however, the [insert number] month rule does apply to one specific sponsor to the same person in this State on the basis of their status as customers of that one specific entity only.

NOTE: The number of months was left blank in this rule because several states currently permit six months; several states allow three months, and other states currently prohibit such periods of enrollment. Whether such enrollment periods should be permissible and the period of time between enrollments are items on which each state should make its decision on an individual basis and each state should modify the time limit in this guideline to comply with the rule adopted by the particular state.

Guideline 15-A(4).

The rule defines the meaning of "a particular insurance product" in Section 15A(2) and prohibits advertising of products having minor variations, such as different elimination periods or different amounts of daily hospital indemnity benefits, in a succession of enrollment periods.

Guideline 16.

The rule is closely related to the requirements of Section 9 concerning the use of statistics. The rule prohibits insurers which have been organized for only a brief period of time advertising that they are "old" and also prohibits the use of illustrations of a "home office" building in a manner which is misleading with respect to the actual size and magnitude of the insurer. Also, the occupations of the persons comprising the insurer's board of directors or the public's familiarity with their names or reputations is irrelevant and must not be emphasized. The preponderance of a particular occupation or profession among the board of directors of an insurer does not justify the advertisement of a plan of insurance offered to the general public as insurance designed or recommended by members of that occupation or profession. For example, it is unacceptable for an insurance company to advertise a policy offered to the general public as "the physicians' policy" or "the doctor's plan" simply because there is a preponderance of physicians or doctors on the board of directors of the insurer. The rule prohibits the use of a recommendation of a commercial rating system unless the purpose, meaning and limitations of the recommendation are clearly indicated.

Guideline 19.

This rule is attached as an example of the text of a rule which may be used at the option of the Commissioner in a state which elects to review advertisements prior to use. The NAIC takes no position here on the question of whether advertising material should be subject to prior review by the Commissioner.

Legislative History (all references are to the <u>Proceedings of the NAIC</u>)

1956 Proc. I 127, 130, 131-137, 148 (adopted).
1956 Proc. II 270, 301, 315 (interpretive guidelines established).
1957 Proc. I 76, 89-90, 99 (amended).
1972 Proc. I 15, 16, 555, 557, 563-580 (amended and reprinted).
1973 Proc. I 9, 11, 141, 224, 244-250 (amended and reprinted).
1973 Proc. II 18, 21, 370, 436, 438-442 (historical notes revised).
1974 Proc. II 8, 10, 380, 419, 420-441 (amended and reprinted).
1989 Proc. I 9, 24-25, 702, 706-726 (amended and reprinted).

Appendix E

DISCLOSURE STATEMENT FOR MEDICARE BENEFICIARIES

Important Notice to Persons on Medicare—This is Not Medicare Supplement Insurance

Some health care services paid for by Medicare may also trigger the payment of benefits under this policy.

This insurance provides limited benefits, if you meet the policy conditions, for hospital or medical expenses only when you are treated for one of the specific diseases or health conditions listed in the policy. It does not pay your Medicare deductibles or coinsurance and is not a substitute for Medicare Supplement insurance.

Medicare generally pays for most or all of these expenses.

Medicare pays extensive benefits for medically necessary services regardless of the reason you need them. These include:

- hospitalization
- physician services
- hospice
- other approved items and services

This policy must pay benefits without regard to other health benefit coverage to which you may be entitled under Medicare or other insurance.

Before You Buy This Insurance

- Check the coverage in **all** health insurance policies you already have.
- For more information about Medicare and Medicare Supplement insurance, review the *Guide to Health Insurance for People with Medicare,* available from the insurance company.
- For help in understanding your health insurance, contact your state insurance department or state senior counseling program.

245

NOTES

1. Health Insurance Association of America. 1996. *Source Book of Health Insurance Data—1995*. Washington, DC: Health Insurance Association of America.
2. Health Insurance Association of America. 1996. *Supplemental Products Survey—1994*. Washington, DC: Health Insurance Association of America.
3. Employee Benefit Research Institute. 1992. *EBRI Data Book on Employee Benefits, 2nd ed.* Washington, DC: Employee Benefit Research Institute.
4. Kerns, Wilmer K. 1994. Protection Against Income Loss During the First 6 Months of Illness or Injury. *Social Security Bulletin* 57 (fall).
5. National Safety Council. 1996. *Accident Facts, 1996 ed*. Itasca, IL: National Safety Council.
6. Couinsky, Kenneth E., et al. 1994. The Impact of Serious Illness on Patients' Families. *Journal of the American Medical Association* 272 (Dec. 21): 1839–1844.
7. American Association of Retired Persons. 1992. *Hospital Indemnity Policy Ownership Among Middle Aged and Older Americans*. Washington, DC: American Association of Retired Persons.
8. Combined Insurance Company of America. 1993. *Policyholder Insurance Ownership and Attitude Research Study*. Chicago, IL: Combined Insurance Company of America.
9. Health Care Financing Administration. Published annually. *Medicare Handbook*. Washington, DC: Health Care Financing Administration, U.S. Department of Health and Human Services.
10. Health Insurance Association of America. 1997. *Source Book of Health Insurance Data, 1996*. Washington, DC: Health Insurance Association of America.
11. Health Care Financing Administration. 1995. *Medicare: A Profile*. Washington, DC: Health Care Financing Administration, U.S. Department of Health and Human Services.

12. Khandker, R.I., and L.A. McCormack. 1996. *Enrollment and Utilization Across Medicare Supplement Plans—Final Report to the Health Care Financing Administration.* Washington, DC: Center for Health Economics Research.

13. Health Care Financing Administration. 1995. *Medicare: A Profile.* Washington, DC: Health Care Financing Administration, U.S. Department of Health and Human Services.

14. Society of Actuaries. 1988. *Individual Health Insurance.* Schaumburg, IL: Society of Actuaries.

15. *Health Insurance Sales Results.* Plainfield, NJ: A.M. Best. August 1996.

16. *Cancer Facts and Figures.* 1993-1996. Atlanta, GA: American Cancer Society, Inc.

17. New York has traditionally rejected the stand-alone concept of specified disease coverage. 11 NYCRR 52.16 provides that "[n]o policy shall provide benefits for specified diseases, or for procedures or treatments unique to specified diseases, and no policy shall provide additional benefits for such specified diseases or procedures, unless the policy also provides insurance which meets the definition contained in sections 52.5, 52.6 or 52.7 of this Part." The referenced code sections refer to basic hospital, basic medical, and major medical coverage.

    Proposed rule 52.15 would reverse this long-standing restriction on stand-alone specified disease coverage. Most of the provisions of the proposed rule are consistent with the regulation of this product in other states. The proposed rule does, however, impose a few unique requirements. Among these requirements are that the policy must provide benefits on an indemnity basis—expense-incurred policies are not allowed. Individuals can only be insured under a total of two specified disease policies, and these two policies must cover different illnesses or diseases. It also prohibits lump-sum diagnosis benefits.

    Connecticut prohibited the sale of specified disease insurance in April 1976 (Public Act 75-616). A series of legislative enactments in 1990 and 1996 reversed this prohibition. In accord with the legislative enactments, the Connecticut Department of Insurance promulgated regulations governing the sale of such policies. These regulations were effective May 31, 1997, and are contained at Section 38(a)505. The

Connecticut regulations are consistent with the regulation of this product across the country, with the exception that group policies are not allowed.

18. Delta Dental Plans Association. 1995. *Facts and Figures: A Report on the Dental Benefits Market, 1994/95.* Chicago, IL: Delta Dental Plans Association.

19. National Association of Dental Plans. 1997. *Managed Dental Care* 3 (Nov.):3.

20. National Center for Health Statistics. 1992. *Vital Health Statistics* 10(183).

21. Health Care Financing Administration. 1996. *Health Care Financing Review* (spring).

22. Foster Higgins. 1995. *National Survey of Employer-Sponsored Health Plans.* New York, NY: Foster Higgins.

23. Health Insurance Association of America. 1997. *Medical Expense Insurance.* Washington, DC: Health Insurance Association of America.

SUGGESTED READINGS

American Council of Life Insurance/Health Insurance Association of America. 1986. *Introduction to Direct Response Marketing in the Life and Health Industry.* Washington, DC: American Council of Life Insurance/Health Insurance Association of America.

Bartleson, E. L. 1974. *Health Insurance Provided Through Individual Policies.* Schaumburg, IL: Society of Actuaries.

Black, K., Jr., and Harold D. Skipper, Jr. 1994. *Life Insurance.* Englewood Cliffs, NJ: Prentice-Hall.

Burgess, Willis W. 1988. Individual Medical Expense Benefits. In *Individual Health Insurance,* edited by Francis T. O'Grady. Schaumburg, IL: Society of Actuaries.

Fagg, Gary. 1986. *Credit Life and Disability Insurance.* Springfield, IL: CLICO Management, Inc.

Hann, Leslie Weirstein. 1996. Indemnity's Last Stand. *Best's Review* (Nov.): 47–52.

Meyer, William F. 1976. *Life and Health Insurance Law, A Summary.* Cincinnati, OH: International Claim Association.

Morrison, Ellen M. 1995. The Path to Health Care Integration. *LIMRA's Market Facts.* (March/April): 23–28.

GLOSSARY

A

ACCIDENT   An unforeseen, unexpected, and unintended event.

ACCIDENT DISABILITY INSURANCE   A type of accident insurance that provides payment to an insured only when the cause of disability is due to an accident.

ACCIDENT INSURANCE   A type of health insurance that insures against loss by accidental bodily injury.

ACCIDENT HOSPITAL INDEMNITY INSURANCE   A type of accident medical insurance that provides payment to an insured or beneficiary for a fixed daily hospital benefit and an accidental death benefit. (See Accident Medical Insurance.)

ACCIDENT MEDICAL INSURANCE   A type of accident insurance that covers medical treatment following an accidental injury; includes hospital, physician, nurse, and laboratory expenses.

ACCIDENTAL BODILY INJURY   An injury sustained as the result of an accident.

ACCIDENTAL DEATH AND DISMEMBERMENT INSURANCE (AD&D)   A form of health and accident insurance that provides payment to an insured's beneficiary in the event of death or the insured in the event of specific bodily losses resulting from an accident.

ACCIDENTAL DEATH BENEFIT   A lump sum payment upon the loss of life of an insured person due to the direct cause of an accident. (See Principal Sum Payment.)

ACCIDENTAL MEANS   The unexpected and unforeseen cause of an accident. The "means" that caused the mishap must be accidental in order to claim benefits under the policy.

ACTIVITIES OF DAILY LIVING (ADL)   Usual activities of an insured in the nonoccupational environment, such as mobility, personal hygiene, dressing, sleeping, and eating. Skills required for community or social living also are included.

ACTUARY Accredited insurance mathematician who calculates premium rates, reserves, and dividends, and who prepares statistical studies and reports.

ADVERSE SELECTION The tendency of those who are poorer-than-average health risks to apply for or maintain insurance coverage. Also called antiselection.

AGENT Insurance company representative licensed by the state who solicits, negotiates, or effects contracts of insurance and who provides services to the policyholder for the insurer.

ALL-CAUSE DEDUCTIBLE A policy provision under which the deductible amount is met by the accumulation of all eligible expenses for any variety of covered claims.

ALLOCATED BENEFITS Benefits for which the maximum amount payable for specific services is itemized in the group contract.

APPROVED AMOUNT Amount Medicare determines is reasonable for a service that is covered under Part B of Medicare. The amount may be less than the actual charge.

ASSOCIATION GROUP INSURANCE A form of group insurance provided to a professional or trade association by which eligible members are covered under one master policy.

ATTAINED-AGE RATE Rate based on the current age of the insured. The rate increases each year as the insured grows older.

AVERAGE WHOLESALE PRICE The published, suggested wholesale price of a drug.

B

BENEFICIARY The person or persons designated by a policyholder to receive insurance policy proceeds.

BENEFICIARY DESIGNATION The person(s) designated to receive accidental death benefits upon the death of an insured.

BENEFIT The amount payable by an insurer to a claimant, assignee, or beneficiary under each coverage in the group contract.

BENEFIT PERIOD (1) The period of time for which benefits are payable under an insurance contract. (2) Method of determining the beneficiary's use of hospital and skilled nursing facility benefits covered by Medicare. It starts when the beneficiary is hospitalized. It ends after the beneficiary has been out of the hospital for 60 days in a row. There is no limit on the number of benefit periods a beneficiary can have.

BENEFIT PROVISION The promises made by the insurer, explained in detail in the contract.

BENEFIT WAITING PERIOD The period of time that must elapse before benefits are payable under a group insurance contract.

BODILY INJURY An injury to the body resulting directly from an accident and independently of all other causes.

BRAND NAME DRUG A medication approved by the FDA for the treatment of a certain medical condition.

BROKER A state-licensed person who places business with several insurers and who represents the insurance buyer rather than the insurance company, even though paid commissions by the insurer.

C

CALENDAR YEAR January 1 through December 31.

CANCER INSURANCE (See Specified Disease Insurance.)

CAPITAL SUM PAYMENT The amount paid under a dismemberment policy for the accidental loss of bodily members.

CARRIER A term sometimes used to identify the party (insurer) to the group contract that agrees to underwrite (carry the risk) and provide certain types of coverage and service.

CIVILIAN HEALTH AND MEDICAL PROGRAM OF THE UNIFORMED SERVICES (CHAMPUS) The organizational mechanisms by which the Department of Defense pays for health care for certain members of the

Uniformed Services through civilian providers; replaced by TRICARE in 1997.

CLAIM A demand to the insurer by, or on behalf of, the insured person for the payment of benefits under a policy.

CLAIMANT Insured or beneficiary exercising the right to receive benefits.

CLASS The category into which insureds are placed in order to determine the amount of coverage for which they are eligible under the policy.

COINSURANCE The arrangement by which the insurer and the insured share a percentage of covered losses after the deductible is met.

COMMISSION The part of an insurance premium an insurer pays an agent or broker for procuring and servicing insurance.

COMMUNITY RATING The process of determining the premium rate for a group risk based wholly or partially on that group's experience.

COORDINATION OF BENEFITS (COB) A method of integrating benefits payable under more than one group health insurance plan so that the insured's benefits from all sources do not exceed 100 percent of allowable medical expenses.

COVERAGE A major classification of benefits provided by a policy (e.g., dental, vision) or the amount of insurance or benefit stated in the policy for which an insured is eligible.

COVERED CHARGES Charges for medical care or supplies that, if incurred by an insured or other covered person, create a liability for the insurer under the terms of a group policy.

COVERED EXPENSES Those specified health care expenses that an insurer will consider for payment under the terms of a health insurance policy.

COVERED PERSON Any person entitled to benefits under a policy (insured or covered dependent).

CREDIT DISABILITY INSURANCE Insurance providing benefits to pay the loan payments if the insured becomes disabled for any cause.

CRITICAL ILLNESS INSURANCE (See Specified Disease Insurance.)

D

DAILY BENEFIT A specified daily maximum amount payable for room and board charges under a hospital indemnity or major medical benefits policy.

DEATH BENEFIT The payment made to a beneficiary at the time of death of an insured.

DEDUCTIBLE The amount of covered expenses that must be incurred and paid by the insured before benefits become payable by the insurer.

DENTAL INSURANCE Insurance providing benefits subject to deductibles, coinsurance, and other policy specifications for expenses incurred in connection with the treatment of dental treatment and diseases. These policies can be integrated into major medical policies or be stand-alone (nonintegrated).

DEPENDENT An insured's spouse (wife or husband), not legally separated from the insured, and unmarried children who meet certain eligibility requirements and who are not otherwise insured under the same group policy. The precise definition of a dependent varies by insurer.

DESIGNATED BENEFICIARY The persons or parties designated by the insured to receive the proceeds of an insurance policy upon the death of the insured.

DIAGNOSIS The determination of the nature and circumstances of a disease condition.

DIAGNOSIS BENEFIT In specified disease insurance, the amount payable by the insurer to a claimant upon diagnosis of the disease or condition covered.

DISABILITY A physical or mental condition that makes an insured incapable of performing one or more duties of his/her own occupation or, for total disability, of any occupation.

DISMEMBERMENT The accidental loss of limb or sight.

DRUG FORMULARY A list of the most commonly prescribed medications that are proven safe and effective in the treatment of certain medical conditions.

E

EFFECTIVE DATE The date that insurance coverage goes into effect.

ELIGIBILITY DATE The date on which a member of an insured group may apply for insurance.

ELIGIBILITY REQUIREMENTS Underwriting requirements the applicant must satisfy in order to become insured.

ELIGIBLE EMPLOYEES Those employees who have met the eligibility requirements for insurance set forth in the group policy.

ELIGIBLE GROUP A group of persons permitted, under state insurance laws and insurer underwriting practices, to be insured under a group policy; usually includes individual employer groups, multiple employer groups, labor union groups, creditor–debtor groups, and certain association groups.

ELIGIBLE MEDICAL EXPENSE A term describing the various types of expense the policy covers. The provision that describes these expenses commonly contains limitations applicable to certain of these expenses.

ELIMINATION PERIOD Period of time after an individual meets the criteria for benefits during which no benefits are payable.

EMPLOYEE-PAY-ALL PLAN A group plan in which the insureds (employees) pay the entire premium.

ENDODONTIC SERVICES Dental services associated with the diagnosis and treatment of diseases of the tooth pulp and areas around the end of the root.

EXCESS CHARGE The difference between the Medicare-approved amount for a service or supply and the actual charge.

EXCLUSIONS (EXCEPTIONS) Specified conditions or circumstances, listed in the policy, for which the policy will not provide benefits.

EXCLUSIVE PROVIDER ORGANIZATIONS (EPO) Form of managed care in which participants are reimbursed for care received only from affiliated providers.

EXPERIENCE RATING The process of determining the premium rate for a group risk based wholly or partially on that risk's experience.

EXTENDED CARE BENEFIT Provides coverage for room and board fees in an extended care facility. Benefits may also include family care, hospice care, and home health care services.

EXTENDED CARE FACILITY A term used to describe an inpatient, nonacute health care facility, such as a nursing home.

F

FEE-FOR-SERVICE A method of charging whereby a physician or other practitioner bills for each visit or service rendered.

FEE SCHEDULE Maximum dollar or unit allowances for health services that apply under a specific contract.

FILING The submission of a proposed policy form for approval to the insurance department of the jurisdiction where it will be issued.

FIRST-DAY COVERAGE A policy that provides coverage from the first day of disability, hospitalization, or medical treatment without elimination periods or deductibles. A characteristic of supplemental plans.

FIRST-DOLLAR COVERAGE A hospital or surgical policy with no deductible amount.

FRANCHISE INSURANCE A form of insurance in which individual policies are issued to the employees of a common employer or the members of an association under an arrangement by which the employer or the members of an association agree to collect premiums and remit them to the insurer.

G

GENERIC DRUG A medication which has the same active ingredients as its brand-name counterpart.

GENERIC SUBSTITUTION A prescription drug plan provision requiring that a generic drug be substituted for a brand name drug when an FDA-approved generic drug is available.

GROUP INSURANCE An arrangement for insuring a number of people under a single, master insurance policy.

GROUP POLICYHOLDER   The legal entity to which the master policy is issued.

GUARANTEED RENEWABLE POLICY   A contract under which an insured has the right, commonly up to a certain age, to continue the policy in force by the timely payment of premiums. However, the insurer reserves the right to change premium rates by policy class.

H

HEALTH INSURANCE   Coverage that provides for the payments of benefits as a result of sickness or injury. Includes insurance for losses from accident, medical expense, disability, or accidental death and dismemberment.

HEALTH MAINTENANCE ORGANIZATION (HMO)   An organization that provides for a wide range of comprehensive health care services for a specified group for a fixed, periodic prepayment.

HOME HEALTH CARE   A comprehensive, medically necessary range of health services provided by a recognized provider organization to a patient at home.

HOSPITAL INDEMNITY INSURANCE   A form of health insurance that provides a stipulated daily, weekly, or monthly payment to an insured during hospital confinement, without regard to the actual expense of the confinement.

HOSPITAL MISCELLANEOUS SERVICES   Services other than room and board and general nursing services provided by a hospital during hospital confinement—such as X-ray examinations, laboratory tests, and medicines.

I

INDEMNITY   A benefit paid by an insurance policy for an insured loss.

INDIVIDUAL INSURANCE   Policies that provide protection to the policyholder and/or his/her family. Sometimes called personal insurance as distinct from group insurance.

IN FORCE The total volume of insurance on the lives of covered employees at any given time (measured in terms of cases, lives, amount [volume] of insurance, or premium).

INJURY Accidental bodily damage sustained while a particular health insurance policy is in force. Coverage excludes underlying health causes or pre-existing conditions that may aggravate or enlarge the loss.

INSURABLE RISK The conditions that make a risk insurable are (a) the peril insured against must produce a definite loss not under the control of the insured, (b) there must be a large number of homogeneous exposures subject to the same perils, (c) the loss must be calculable and the cost of insuring it must be economically feasible, (d) the peril must be unlikely to affect all insureds simultaneously, and (e) the loss produced by a risk must be definite and have a potential to be financially serious.

INSURANCE A plan of risk management that, for a price, offers the insured an opportunity to share the costs of possible economic loss through an entity called an insurer.

INSURANCE COMPANY Any corporation primarily engaged in the business of furnishing insurance protection to the public.

INSURED The person (employee, dependent, or group member) who is covered for insurance under the group policy and to whom, or on behalf of whom, the insurer agrees to pay benefits.

INSURER The party to the insurance contract that promises to pay losses or benefits. Also, any corporation primarily engaged in the business of furnishing insurance protection to the public.

INTEGRATED PLAN A supplemental plan (e.g., dental) integrated with other medical expense coverage.

ISSUE-AGE RATE Rate based on the age of the insured at the time the premium is purchased. The rate does not increase as insured gets older.

J

JOINT BENEFICIARY Person or party legally entitled to share in the proceeds of an insurance policy.

L

LIMITATION   A provision that sets a cap on specific coverage.

LIMITED POLICY   Policy that covers only specified accidents or sicknesses.

LIMITING CHARGE   The maximum amount a physician may charge a beneficiary for a covered service if the physician does not accept Medicare assignment. The limit is 15 percent above the fee schedule for nonparticipating physicians.

LONG-TERM CARE   A wide range of health and personal care—from simple assisted living arrangements to intensive nursing home care—for elderly or disabled persons.

LOSS   (1) The amount of insurance or benefit for which the insurer becomes liable when the event insured against occurs; (2) the happening of the event insured against.

LOSS RATIO   The ratio of incurred claims to premiums (incurred claims divided by earned premiums).

LUMP SUM PAYMENT   The full amount paid as a single sum upon the initial diagnosis of an insured under a specified disease policy.

M

MAIL-ORDER PHARMACY   A method of dispensing medication directly to the insured through the mail by means of a mail-order drug distribution company.

MAJOR MEDICAL EXPENSE INSURANCE   A form of health insurance that provides benefits for most types of medical expense up to a high maximum benefit. Such contracts may contain internal limits and usually are subject to deductibles and coinsurance.

MANAGED CARE   The term used to describe the coordination of financing and provision of health care to produce high-quality health care on a cost-effective basis.

MANDATED BENEFITS   Certain coverages required by state law to be included in health insurance contracts.

MAXIMUM ALLOWABLE COST (MAC) The maximum dollar amount a pharmacy is paid for a particular generic drug.

MAXIMUM BENEFIT The maximum length of time for which benefits are payable during any one period of disability.

MAXIMUM BENEFIT PERIOD The highest amount any one individual may receive under an insurance contract.

MAXIMUM DAILY HOSPITAL BENEFIT The maximum amount payable for hospital room and board per day of hospital confinement.

MEDICAL EVENT BENEFIT In specified disease insurance, the amount payable by the insurer to a claimant when the insured has a medical event common to the treatment of the covered illness or disease. Medical events include inpatient benefits, surgical procedures, nonsurgical procedures, and extended care.

MEDICAL SAVINGS ACCOUNT (MSA) A trust or custodial account created to pay the qualified medical expenses of the account holder. Provides tax-favored treatment of out-of-pocket medical expenses.

MEDICARE A federally sponsored program that provides hospital benefits, supplementary medical care, and catastrophic coverages to persons aged 65 and older and to some other eligibles.

MEDICARE ASSIGNMENT Arrangement whereby the physician (or medical supplier) agrees to accept the Medicare-approved amount as full payment for services and supplies covered under Part B of Medicare.

MEDICARE+CHOICE Medicare Part C, a private Medicare health plan system that includes the traditional Medicare fee-for-service program, coordinated health plans including HMOs and PPOs, and a private fee-for-service supplemental plan. Available to individuals entitled to Medicare Part A and enrolled in Part B.

MEDICARE HOSPITAL INSURANCE Part A of Medicare. Helps pay for medically necessary care in a hospital, skilled nursing facility, or psychiatric hospital and for hospice and home health care.

MEDICARE MEDICAL INSURANCE Part B of Medicare. Helps pay for medically necessary physician services and other medical services and supplies not covered by Part A.

MEDICARE PART C   A private Medicare health plan system, Medicare+Choice, established by the Balanced Budget Act. Includes the traditional Medicare fee-for-service program, coordinated health plans including HMOs and PPOs, and a private fee-for-service supplemental plan. See also Medicare+Choice.

MEDICARE SELECT   The same as a standard Medicare supplement plan except specific hospitals and, in some cases, physicians must be used, except in an emergency, to be eligible for full benefits.

MEDIGAP   Term applied to private insurance products that supplement federal insurance benefits under Medicare. Also called MedSup.

MISCELLANEOUS EXPENSE   Expenses connected with hospital insurance; hospital charges other than room and board, such as X-rays, drugs, laboratory fees, and other ancillary charges.

MISCELLANEOUS HOSPITAL EXPENSE BENEFIT   A policy provision that provides benefits for expenses for necessary hospital services and supplies, such as X-rays, laboratory tests, medicines, surgical dressings, anesthetics, and use of an operating room.

MORBIDITY   The frequency and severity of sicknesses and accidents in a well-defined class or classes of persons.

MORTALITY   The death rate in a group of people as determined from prior experience.

N

NATIONAL ASSOCIATION OF INSURANCE COMMISSIONERS (NAIC)   A national organization of state officials who are charged with the regulation of insurance. The association was formed to promote national uniformity in the regulation of insurance. It has no official power but wields tremendous influence.

NONCANCELLABLE POLICY   A contract the insured can continue in force by the timely payment of the set premium until at least age 50 or, in the case of a policy issued after age 44, for at least five years from its date of issue. The insurer may not unilaterally change any contract provision of the in-force policy, including premium rates.

NONINTEGRATED PLAN A supplemental plan (e.g., dental) written separately (not integrated) from other coverages.

NONMEDICAL-RELATED EXPENSES Significant expenses associated with serious illness or disease that are not directly related to the provision of medical care and covered under some specified disease policies (e.g., travel to receive appropriate treatment, special diets, loss of income, child care).

NONOCCUPATIONAL INSURANCE Insurance that does not provide benefits for an accident or sickness arising out of a person's employment.

NONRENEWABLE POLICY A policy issued for a single term that is designed to cover the insured during a period of short-term risk.

NOTICE OF CLAIM A written notice to the insurer by an insured claiming a covered loss.

O

OCCUPATIONAL RATE A variation in premium based upon occupational class, due to differences among occupations in the incidence of accidents or illness.

OPEN ENROLLMENT A time during which uninsured employees and/or their dependents may obtain coverage under an existing group plan, and Medicare beneficiaries may obtain coverage from any Medicare supplement plan, without presenting evidence of insurability. Differs from a resolicitation in that a minimum number of applications are not required.

OPTIONALLY RENEWABLE POLICY A contract of health insurance under which the insurer has the right to terminate the coverage at any policy anniversary or, in some cases, at any premium due date.

ORAL SURGICAL SERVICES Dental services associated with the diagnosis and surgical management of oral diseases, injuries, and defects of the jaw. Technically, any cutting procedure in the oral cavity.

ORTHODONTIC SERVICES Dental services associated with the preventive and corrective treatment for irregularities in the alignment of the teeth.

OUT-OF-POCKET EXPENSE Those medical expenses that an insured must pay that are not covered under the group contract.

OVER-THE-COUNTER (OTC) DRUG An FDA-approved medication that is thought to be safe and effective for self-medication. An OTC drug is available without a prescription.

P

PARTICIPATING PHYSICIAN A physician or medical supplier who agrees to accept assignment on all Medicare claims.

PATENT An exclusive right to produce a product for a number of years.

PER CAUSE DEDUCTIBLE The flat amount that the insured must pay toward the eligible medical expenses resulting from each illness before the insurance company will make any benefit payments.

PER DIEM COST Literally, cost per day. Refers in general to hospital or other inpatient institutional costs per day or for a day of care. Per diem costs are averages and do not reflect true costs for each patient.

PERIODONTIC SERVICES Dental services associated with the prevention, diagnosis, and treatment of diseases of the structures commonly referred to as the gums that surround and support the teeth.

PHARMACY PROVIDER NETWORK A group of pharmacies that contract with a health care plan to fill prescription drug orders for insureds at agreed-upon rates.

POINT-OF-SERVICE (POS) PROGRAM Health care delivery method offered as an option of an employer's indemnity program. Under such a program, employees coordinate their health care needs through a primary care physician.

POLICY The document that sets forth the contract of insurance.

POLICYHOLDER The legal entity to whom an insurer issues a contract.

PORTABILITY Quality of an insurance policy that is designed to allow an insured employee to accumulate and transfer insurance benefits from one employer to another, or from an employer to a nongroup or personal policy.

PRE-EXISTING CONDITION   A mental or physical problem suffered by an insured prior to the effective date of insurance coverage.

PRE-EXISTING CONDITIONS PROVISION   A restriction on payments for those charges directly resulting from an accident or illness for which the insured received care or treatment within a specified period of time (e.g., three months) prior to the date of insurance.

PREFERRED PROVIDER ORGANIZATION (PPO)   A managed care arrangement consisting of a group of hospitals, physicians, and other providers who have contracts with an insurer, employer, third-party administrator, or other sponsoring group to provide health care services to covered persons.

PREMIUM   The amount paid an insurer for specific insurance protection.

PREMIUM RATE   The price of a unit of coverage or benefit.

PRESCRIPTION DRUG   Any medication or medicinal substance that is approved by the Food and Drug Administration (FDA) and can only be dispensed only according to a prescription drug order, under federal or state law.

PRESCRIPTION DRUG ORDER   A request for a prescription drug by a physician (or other health care practitioner) licensed to prescribe medications by the state.

PRESCRIPTION DRUG PLAN   A provision in some health plans that allows insureds to obtain prescription drugs without incurring potentially large out-of-pocket expenses.

PREVENTIVE SERVICES   Services designed to prevent or promote early detection of specified diseases or conditions. In dental insurance, professional cleaning of teeth and fluoride treatments. In cancer insurance, mammography, colonoscopy, and other tests.

PRIMARY BENEFICIARY   The first person(s) designated to receive the proceeds of an insurance policy upon death of the insured.

PRINCIPAL SUM PAYMENT The amount paid in one sum in event of accidental death and, in some cases, accidental dismemberment.

PROGRESSIVE PAYMENT An increase in the amount of a diagnosis benefit paid in some specified disease policies based on the length of time the insured has been covered under the policy.

PROOF OF LOSS Documentary evidence required by an insurer to prove that a valid claim exists, usually consisting of a claim form completed by the insured and the insured's attending physician.

PROSTHODONTIC SERVICES Dental services associatd with replacing missing natural teeth and tissues with a device or appliance.

PROVIDER-SPONSORED ORGANIZATION (PSO) Used by doctors and hospitals to directly contract with Medicare. A public, private entity established or organized and operated by a health care provider, or group of affiliated providers, that offers a substantial proportion of health care items and services under a HCFA contract, directly through the provider or affiliated group of providers, and that shares substantial risk, directly or indirectly, with respect to the provision of such items and services and has at least a majority financial interest in the entity.

PROVISION A part of an insurance contract that describes or explains a feature, benefit, condition, or requirement of the insurance protection afforded by the contract.

R

RATING Determining the cost of a given unit of insurance for a given year.

REASONABLE AND CUSTOMARY CHARGE (See Usual and Customary Charge.)

REIMBURSEMENT An amount paid to an insured for expenses actually incurred as a result of an accident or sickness. Payment will not exceed the amount specified in the policy.

RESTORATIVE SERVICES Dental services associated with the repair or restoration of teeth due to caries (cavities), trauma, impaired function, abrasion, or erosion.

GLOSSARY

RIDER A document that modifies or amends the insurance contract.

RISK The probable amount of loss foreseen by an insurer in issuing a contract. The term sometimes also applies to the person insured or to the hazard insured against.

S

SCHEDULE A listing of amounts payable for specified occurrences (e.g., surgical operations, laboratory tests, X-ray services, and such).

SCHEDULE OF INSURANCE A list of the amounts of insurance per person for each coverage according to predetermined classifications, decided on by the policyholder and insurer.

SPECIFIED DISEASE INSURANCE Insurance providing an unallocated benefit, subject to a maximum amount, for expenses incurred in connection with the treatment of specified diseases, such as cancer and other critical illnesses. These policies are designed to supplement major medical policies.

STATE INSURANCE DEPARTMENT An administrative agency that implements state insurance laws and supervises (within the scope of these laws) the activities of insurers operating within the state.

SUPPLEMENTAL HEALTH INSURANCE Health insurance policies that fill in the gaps of medical expense coverages (e.g., deductibles, coinsurance, and maximum out-of-pocket expenses); provide additional benefits (e.g., dental, prescription drugs, and vision care); and cover additional expenses as a result of a severe accident or illness (e.g., accident medical expenses).

T

TRAVEL ACCIDENT POLICIES A type of travel accident insurance that covers accidents that occur while an insured person is traveling on business for an employer, away from the usual place of business and only on named conveyances, including scheduled airlines, other common carriers (including taxis, buses, and subways), and motor vehicle accidents. Can be one-trip or multiple-trip coverage.

TRICARE The organizational mechanisms by which the Department of Defense pays for health care for certain members of the Uniformed Services through civilian providers; replaced CHAMPUS in 1997.

24-HOUR COVERAGE Insurance providing benefits at any time for an accident or sickness incurred either on or off the job.

U

UNDERWRITER The term generally applies to (a) a company that receives the premiums and accepts responsibility for the fulfillment of the policy contract, (b) the company employee who decides whether or not the company should assume a particular risk, or (c) the agent who sells the policy.

UNDERWRITING The process by which an insurer determines whether or not and on what basis it will accept an application for insurance.

UNIFORM PREMIUM A rating structure in which one premium applies to all insureds, regardless of age, sex, or occupation.

USUAL AND CUSTOMARY CHARGE A charge for health care that is consistent with the average rate or charge for identical or similar services in a certain geographic area.

V

VISION PLAN A provision in some health plans that provides vision and eye health care.

W

WAITING PERIOD A specified number of days at policy inception during which the insured must remain healthy or no benefits are payable under the policy. Used in specified disease insurance.

WAIVER The voluntary surrender of a right or privilege known to exist.

WAIVER (EXCLUSION ENDORSEMENT) An agreement attached to the policy and accepted by the insured that eliminates a specified pre-existing physical condition or specified hazard from coverage under the policy.

WELLNESS BENEFIT In specified disease insurance, the amount payable by the insurer to a claimant, usually a flat fee, after a covered test is performed. Designed to encourage prevention or early detection of the serious illness covered by the insurance.

WORKERS' COMPENSATION Liability insurance requiring certain employers to pay benefits and furnish medical care to employees for on-the-job injuries, and to pay benefits to dependents of employees killed by occupational accidents.

INDEX

Accident, 180
Accidental death (AD), 73, 101, 105, 109
Accidental death and dismemberment (AD&D) insurance, 23, 105-106, 110-111, 187
Accidental injury, 101, 102-103, 180
Accidental means, 101-102, 180
Accidental result, 102
Accident and sickness insurance, 171, 221-222
Accident disability insurance, 12, 23, 106-107, 109, 111-112
Accident hospital indemnity policy (AHIP), 23, 104-105, 110
Accident insurance policies, 101-122
  dental insurance, 129-130
Accident medical expense insurance, 4, 22, 104, 110
Accident-only coverage, 188, 191, 208
Accidents, 102-103
Administrative procedures, 175, 217
Adverse selection, hospital indemnity policy, 76, 77-78
  see also Antiselection
Advertising, 217, 220-221, 223-243
  accident medical expense policies, 120-121
  benefits payable, losses covered or premiums payable, 223-225
  form and content, 223
  interpretive guidelines, 232-243
  specified disease insurance, 97-98
Age distribution, hospital indemnity policy, 78
Age-banded rates
  hospital indemnity policy, 75, 78
  Medicare supplement plans, 53
Agents, 3
  accident medical expense policies, 109
  hospital indemnity policy, 68, 69, 70, 76
  Medicare supplement plans, 37
  specified disease insurance, 88, 89
  supplemental insurance, 3
  see also Brokers
AIDS, specified disease insurance, 93, 97
All-accident policy, 105
All-cause deductible, specified disease insurance, 84
Anesthesia services, 189, 190
Antiselection, 16
  hospital indemnity policy, 78
  see also Adverse selection
Any willing pharmacy provider, 160
Applicability and scope, 214
Applicant, 213
Application, accident medical expense policies, 114
Application forms, 210
Associations
  Medicare supplement plans, 38, 55
  specified disease insurance, 88
Attained-age rating
  accident medical expense policies, 118
  Medicare supplement plans, 53
Automated services, hospital indemnity policy, 70
Automobile/pedestrian benefits, accident medical expense policies, 111
Average wholesale price (AWP), 155

Balanced Budget Act of 1997, 30, 57
Banks, supplemental health insurance and, 168
Basic coverage, 5
Basic hospital and medical-surgical expense coverage, 203-204
Basic hospital expense coverage, 188-189, 201-202
Basic medical-surgical expense coverage, 189, 202-203
Basic services, dental insurance, 129, 130
Beneficiary, 47, 57
Benefit period
  hospital indemnity policy, 72
  Medicare, 31, 33, 35
Benefits
  accident medical expense policies, 109-113
  coordination, 19
  dental insurance, 127-138
  hospital indemnity policy, 71-75
  limits, specified disease insurance, 85
  maximums, specified disease insurance, 85
  Medicare supplement plans, 39-45
  specified disease insurance, 89-92
Benefit triggers, specified disease insurance, 89, 91
Billing vehicle, hospital indemnity policy, 69
Bodily injury, 101-102
Brand-name drug, 151
Broad market, hospital indemnity policy, 69
Brokers
  hospital indemnity policy, 68
  specified disease insurance, 89
  see also Agents
Building benefit, specified disease insurance, 92

Buyer's Guide, specified disease insurance, 97

Calendar year, 33, 36
Cancellability, 226
Cancer insurance, 21, 83, 90, 92, 96, 97, 192, 194-198
Certificate, 213, 222
Certificate form, 213
CHAMPUS, 26, 145, 162
Charge limitation, Medicare supplement plans, 46
Child care, specified disease insurance, 87
Claims processing, on-line, prescription drugs, 155-156
Clinical diagnosis
Coinsurance
  hospital indemnity policy, 64, 65
  Medicare, 31, 32
  specified disease insurance, 85
Commissions, Medicare supplement plans, 37, 58-59
Common carrier coverage, accident medical expense policies, 107-108
Community rated
  accident medical expense policies, 118
  Medicare supplement plans, 54
Comprehensive medical insurance plans, gaps, 84
Convalescence, 187
Convalescent nursing home, 179-180
Copayments
  hospital indemnity policy, 65
  prescription drugs, 149-150
  specified disease insurance, 85
Cosmetic surgery, 184
Cost-based plan, Medicare supplement plans, 49

INDEX

Cost management, supplemental health insurance and, 166
Cost sharing, prescription drugs, 150
Credit disability insurance, accident medical expense policies, 107
Critical illness coverage, 21-22, 83, 84
Crowns, 134
Customer service
　hospital indemnity policy, 70
　Medicare supplement plans, 38-39
　specified disease insurance, 88-89

Daily room and board hospital benefit, 71-72, 188, 190
Data collection, supplemental health insurance and, 167-168
Death due to covered disease, specified disease insurance, 92
Deceptive words, phrases or illustrations, 223-225
Deductibles
　accident medical expense policies, 104
　hospital indemnity policy, 64-65
　Medicare, 31, 32
　prescription drugs, 150
　specified disease insurance, 84-85
Defined contribution, 167
Demographic factors, dental insurance, 142
Dental care costs, 125, 185
Dental disease, 123
Dental insurance, 4, 7, 9, 24, 123-144
　annual premium, 4
　by employer size, 126
　covered charges, 126-127
　plans, 127-128
Dental services, frequency, 130, 131
Dependents, accident medical expense policies, 104

Diagnosis
　dental insurance, 131
　specified disease insurance, 91
Direct solicitation, specified disease insurance, 88
Disability, short-term, 67
Disability income insurance, 11-12, 183, 187, 191, 207
Disclosure, 174, 216
　accident medical expense policies, 119
　hospital indemnity policy, 79
　Medicare beneficiaries, 245
　Medicare supplement plans, 59
　method, 223
　provisions, 198-210
　specified disease insurance, 94-95
　specified disease insurance, 96-97
Discounts, Medicare supplement plans, 55
Disease state management, prescription drugs, 157
Dismemberment, 188
Disparaging comparisons and statements, 228
Dispense as written (DAW), prescription drugs, 152
Dispensing fee, 155
Distribution
　accident medical expense policies, 109
　Medicare supplement plans, 37
　specified disease insurance, 87-88
　supplemental health insurance and, 168, 169
Dividend policy, 183
Drug formulary, 153-154

Education, supplemental insurance purchaser, 15
Effective date, 217

275

Electronic claims, 39
Elimination period, accident medical expense policies, 104, 113
Employee benefits, supplemental health insurance and, 166-167
Employers
  benefits, 5-6
  Medicare supplement plans, 38
End-stage renal disease, 37, 51
Endodontic services, dental insurance, 137
Endorsed market, hospital indemnity policy, 69
Endorsements, 226-227
Enforcement procedures, 231
Enrollment, accident medical expense policies, 114
Enrollment form
Examinations, dental insurance, 131
Excepted benefits, specified disease insurance, 95
Exceptions, 222, 225
Exceptions and limitations
  accident medical expense policies, 112-113
  dental insurance, 130
  Medicare supplement plans, 45-46
  prescription drugs, 152-153
  specified disease insurance, 85-86, 92
Exclusions
  accident medical expense policies, 111
  hospital indemnity policy, 75
Exclusive provider organizations (EPOs), dental insurance, 127
Expenses, hospital indemnity policy, 77
Extended care
  facility, 179-180
  specified disease insurance, 91
Extractions, 135

Family coverage, 186, 187
Federal regulations
  accident medical expense policies, 119
  dental insurance, 143
  hospital indemnity policy, 78-79
  prescription drugs, 159
  specified disease insurance, 94-95
Fee-for-service indemnity plans, dental insurance, 127
Filing for prior review, 231-232
Filing requirements for advertisement, 217
Fillings, 133
Financial incentives, pharmacists, 158
First-day coverage, 22, 31, 71-72
Food and Drug Administration (FDA), 151
Foot care, 184
Form, 171
Format, 174

Generic drug, 151-152
Generic substitution, 152
Group or quasi-group implications, 229-230
Guaranteed issue
  accident medical expense policies, 114
  hospital indemnity policy, 76, 77
  Medicare supplement plans, 51, 57
Guaranteed rate, accident medical expense policies, 114
Guaranteed renewable, 18, 114, 186, 192

Health Care Financing Administration (HCFA), 30
Health care coverages, 1-2, 5
Health Insurance for the Aged Act, 182-183

INDEX

Health Insurance Portability and Accountability Act of 1996 (HIPAA), 95, 79, 119
Health maintenance organizations (HMOs), 166
  dental insurance, 128
  hospital indemnity policy, 64
  Medicare and, 47-50
  see also, Medicare SELECT
Heart attack, hospital indemnity policy, 73
Heart surgery, 8-9
Hospital, 178-179
Hospital confinement indemnity coverage, 184, 189, 205
Hospital indemnity insurance, 11, 12, 20-21
Hospital indemnity policy (HIP), 63-81
Human immunodeficiency virus (HIV), specified disease insurance, 93, 97

Identification of plan or number of policies, 227
Identity of insurer, 228-229
Income replacement supplements, 11-12, 14
Individual coverage, 6, 200-201
Indivudual Accident and Sickness Insurance Minimum Standards Act, 171-175
Inhospital medical services, 189, 190
Injury, 180
Inlays, 133
Inpatient benefits, specified disease insurance, 90
Institutional advertisement, 222
Insurer, 222
Integrated plans, 24
  dental insurance, 128

Intensive care, hospital indemnity policy, 72
Internal benefit limit, hospital indemnity policy, 66
Internet, supplemental health insurance and, 168
Introductory, initial, or special offers, 230-231
Invitation to contract, 222
Invitation to inquire, 222
Issue-age rating
  accident medical expense policies, 117-118
  Medicare supplement plans, 53-54
Issuer, 213

Jurisdictional licensing and status of insurer, 228

Kidney failure, 8, 29
  see also End-stage renal disease

Lead-generating device, 222-223
Limitations, 184-185, 222, 225
  new dental insurance plans, 139-140
Limited benefit plans, 146-147, 209-210
Lodging, specified disease insurance, 86
Loss of life, accident medical expense policies, 111
Loss of limb, accident medical expense policies, 111
Loss ratio, 167
  Medicare supplement plans, 38, 58
  standards, 216
Lost income, 6, 9
  specified disease insurance, 87

277

Lump sum
  accident medical expense policies, 118
  indemnity coverage, 197
  specified disease insurance, 91, 92

Mail-order pharmacy, 156
  equity, 160
Maintenance drug, 149
Major medical expense coverage, 189-191, 205-207
Major medical plan, 63
Major services, dental insurance, 129, 130
Managed care, 5, 166
Mandated benefits, 160-161
Marketing standards, Medicare supplement plans, 59-60
Mass marketing
  accident medical expense policies, 109
  hospital indemnity policy, 68-69, 76
  Medicare supplement plans, 38
  specified disease insurance, 88, 97
  supplemental health insurance and, 3, 167-168
Massachusetts, specified disease insurance, 99
Maternity benefits
  hospital indemnity policy, 74-75
  see also Pregnancy
Maximum allowable cost (MAC), prescription drugs, 152
Maximum benefit limits
  accident medical expense policies, 110-111, 112, 115-116
  prescription drugs, 150
Maximum out-of-pocket expenses, hospital indemnity policy, 65-66

Meals and special diets, specified disease insurance, 86
Medical event benefits, specified disease insurance, 90
Medical expenses, 6, 7-9
  specified disease insurance, 84
Medical savings accounts (MSAs), 31
  dental insurance, 143
Medicare, 29-32, 182-183, 213
  beneficiary satisfaction, 31, 32
  enrollment, 29
  Part A, 29, 30, 31, 32, 34, 35
  Part B, 29, 30, 33-34, 36-37
  Part C, 30
  qualification, 58
  risk, 48, 58
  specified disease insurance and, 94
Medicare+Choice, 30-31, 49
  enrollment procedures, 50-51
  licensing, 57
  qualification, 58
  supplemental health insurance and, 167
Medicare SELECT, 7, 46-47, 58
Medicare supplement insurance, 4, 7, 8, 15, 16, 19-20, 29-61, 213-214
  annual premium, 4
  Plan A, 39-41
  Plan B, 40, 41
  Plan D, 40, 41-42
  Plan E, 40, 42
  Plan F, 40, 42-43
  Plan G, 40, 43
  Plan H, 40, 43-44
  Plan I, 40, 44
  Plan J, 40, 44-45
  plans, 20
  short-term, 7-8
  standardization, 56, 60-61
  supplemental health insurance and, 167

Medicare Supplement Insurance Minimum Standards Model Act, 56, 213–217
Medigap, 29, 58
MedSup, 29
Melanoma. *See* Skin cancer
Mental disorder, 183, 184
 hospital indemnity policy, 74
Military service exclusion, 187
Minimum benefit requirements, specified disease insurance, 96
Minimum benefits standard, 173, 185–198
 cancer coverage, 196–197
 lump-sum indemnity coverage, 197–198
 specified disease coverage, 193–194
Miscellaneous hospital services, 188, 190
Modal discount, Medicare supplement plans, 55
Model Regulation to Implement the Individual Accident and Sickness Insurance Minimum Standards Act, 177–212
Model regulation, 55–56, 59–60
Monthly income, accident medical expense policies, 106–107, 111–112

National Association of Insurance Commissioners (NAIC), 80
 advertising guidelines, specified disease insurance, 97–98
 authority, 177
 Model Regulation to Implement the Individual Accident and Sickness Insurance Minimum Standards Act, 177–212
 Minimum Standards Act, specified disease insurance, 96–97
 supplemental health insurance and, 167
Nervous disorder. *See* Mental disorder
New Jersey, specified disease insurance, 98–99
Noncancellable, 18, 186
 accident medical expense policies, 114
Noncovered expenses
 hospital indemnity policy, 65
 Medicare, 34, 37
 see also Related expenses
Nonintegrated plans, 24–25
 dental insurance, 128–129
Nonmedical expenses, 10
Nonoccupational coverage, 23
 accident medical expense policies, 106
Nonscheduled plan, dental insurance, 129
Nonsmoker discount, Medicare supplement plans, 55
Nonsurgical treatment, specified disease insurance, 91
Notice of free examination, 217
Nurse, 181

Occupation, supplemental insurance purchaser, 15
Occupational classifications, accident medical expense policies, 116
Omnibus Budget Reconciliation Act (OBRA), 47, 55, 79, 94–95, 119
One period of confinement, 178
One trip/multiple trips, accident medical expense policies, 108
Onlays, 134
Open enrollment, Medicare supplement plans, 49, 51, 57, 61

279

Optional benefits, hospital indemnity policy, 73
Oral surgery, dental insurance, 135-136
Orthodontic services, dental insurance, 137-138
Out-of-hospital care, 190
Out-of-pocket costs, 165
  dental insurance, 125
Outpatient medical expenses, 73
Outpatient services, 188
Over-the-counter (OTC) drug, 152
Overall maximums, specified disease insurance, 85
Ownership, 19

Partial disability, 182
Patent, prescription drugs, 151
Pathological diagnosis, specified disease insurance, 91
Payroll deductions
  hospital indemnity policy, 68
  specified disease insurance, 87
  supplemental health insurance and, 168
Penaltics, 217
Per-cause deductible, specified disease insurance, 85
Periodontic services, dental insurance, 136-137
Person, 222
Pharmacy benefit manager (PBM), 154-156
Pharmacy network management, 155
Pharmacy payment, 155
Pharmacy provider network, 155
Pharmacy standards, 155
Physician, 181
Point-of-service (POS) option, Medicare supplement plans, 48

Policy, 171, 120, 214
Polio, specified disease insurance, 83, 99
Portability, dental insurance, 143
Pre-existing conditions, 16-17, 174-175, 181, 183, 184, 225
  dental insurance, 140
  hospital indemnity policy, 73-74, 74-75
  Medicare supplement plans, 45-46, 52, 57, 60
  NAIC, 16
  specified disease insurance, 92
Preferred provider organizations (PPOs), dental insurance, 127
Pregnancy, 184, 187
  see also Maternity benefits
Premiums, 17-18
  credit, Medicare supplement plans, 58
  dental insurance, 141
  hospital indemnity policy, 70-71
  increases, Medicare supplement plans, 54
  Medicare supplements, 39
  stability, 17
Prepayment plans, dental insurance, 123
Prescription drug, covered, 151-152
Prescription drug insurance, 9, 25
Prescription drug order, 151
Prescription drug plan, 145, 148-161
Preventive services, dental insurance, 124, 132-133, 138
Pricing, hospital indemnity policy, 77, 78
Principal sum, 105
Prior dental coverage, dental insurance, 141-142
Progressive payment, specified disease insurance, 92

Prohibited policy provision, 183
Prosthodontic services, dental insurance, 134-135
Provider-sponsored organization (PSO), 57
Purchaser, 14-15

Quality assessment, prescription drugs, 157-158

Railway travelers, 101
Rate classes, 18-19
Rate review standards, hospital indemnity policy, 80-81
Rating
  accident medical expense policies, 117-118
  dental insurance, 140-142
  hospital indemnity policy, 77-78
  Medicare supplement plans, 52-55
  prescription drugs, 159
  specified disease insurance, 93-94
Recovery time, hospital indemnity policy, 73
Recurrent disabilities, 187
Reductions, 222, 225
Referral discount plans, dental insurance, 128
Refunds, Medicare supplement plans, 58
Regulations
  accident medical expense policies, 119-121
  dental insurance, 143
  hospital indemnity policy, 78-81
  limited benefit plans, 147
  Medicare supplement plans, 55-60
  prescription drugs, 159-160
  specified disease insurance, 94-99

Reimbursement percentage, specified disease insurance, 85
Reimbursement plans, prescription drugs, 25, 149
Related expenses, 6, 9-13
  hospital indemnity policy, 67-68
  see also, Noncovered expenses
Related expenses, specified disease insurance, 86-87
Renewability, 226
Renewability options, accident medical expense policies, 114
Requirements for replacement, 210-212
Residual disability, 182
Restorative services, dental insurance, 133-134
Retail pharmacy equity, 160
Rider, 183
  accident medical expense policies, 110
  hospital indemnity policy, 72
Risk-based plan, Medicare supplement plans, 48-49
Risk classification, 167
Risk selection factors, specified disease insurance, 93
Rules Governing Advertisements of Accident and Sickness Insurance with Interpretive Guidelines, 219-243

Sales restrictions and limitations, specified disease insurance, 98-99
Scheduled plan, dental insurance, 128
Selective underwriting, Medicare supplement plans, 51-52
Separability, 212, 217
Service plans, prescription drugs, 25, 149-150

Severability provision, 231
Sex distribution, hospital indemnity policy, 78
Short-form application, accident medical expense policies, 115
Sick leave, 11, 67
Sickness, 180-181
Skilled nursing facility, 31, 179-180
Skilled nursing home, 197
Skin cancer, specified disease insurance, 92, 93
Small employer market reforms, specified disease insurance, 98
Social Security Act, 29
Specialty plans, 25-26, 145-164
Specialty risk products, 83
Specified accident coverage, 198
Specified diseases, 83-84
Specified disease and specified accident coverage, 173, 192-198, 208-209
Specified disease insurance, 5, 21-22, 83-100
  annual premium, 5
Sports/sporting events, accident medical expense policies, 105, 116
Spousal discount, Medicare supplement plans, 55
Standards for policy provisions, 172-173
Standards for policy provisions and authority to promulgate regulations, 214-215
State regulations
  accident medical expense policies, 120
  dental insurance, 143
  hospital indemnity policy, 79-80
  prescription drugs, 159-160
  specified disease insurance, 95-99
Statement about an insurer, 231
Statistics, 227

Student/sports accident policies, 105, 116
Supplement, 1
Supplemental health insurance, 1-2, 6
  annual premium, 4
  classification, 5-13
  market, 1, 2-5, 165-169
Surgery benefits, hospital indemnity policy, 73
Surgical services, 189, 190
  specified disease insurance, 91

Telemarketing, accident medical expense policies, 109
Termination of policy, 188, 226
Testimonials, 226-227
Therapeutic substitution, 153
Time limits, 174
Tooth extraction, 136
Total disability, 181-182
Travel
  other than common carrier, accident medical expense policies, 108
  specified disease insurance, 86
Travel accident insurance, 23-24, 106, 107-108, 112
Treatment, high-cost, 8-9
TRICARE supplement, 25, 26, 145, 162-163
Trip cancellation
24-hour accident policy, 23, 105, 106
Twisting, 60

Underwriting, 15-16
  accident medical expense policies, 113-117
  dental insurance, 138-140
  hospital indemnity policy, 76-77
  Medicare supplement plans, 51-52

prescription drugs, 158
specified disease insurance, 93
Unintentional injury, 103
Usual and customary charges, hospital indemnity policy, 64, 66-67

Veneers, 134
Vision insurance, 7, 9, 25-26, 161, 185
Voluntary plans, dental insurance, 128, 144

Waiting period, 92, 183
Waivers, 185
Wellness benefits, specified disease insurance, 89-90
Workers' compensation
Workplace, supplemental insurance, 3

X-rays, dental insurance, 132